ESOPHAGUS ATTACK!

ESOPHAGUS
ATTACK!

THE 3-STEP METHOD TO ENJOY EATING AGAIN

DOUG LAKE, MD

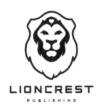

LIONCREST
PUBLISHING

ESOPHAGUS ATTACK!

The 3-Step Method to Enjoy Eating Again

ISBN   978-1-5445-1698-1   *Hardcover*

978-1-5445-1697-4   *Paperback*

978-1-5445-1696-7   *Ebook*

To Maleia, Grace, Charlotte, and Caroline. Your
unending love amazes me.

To Mom and Dad. Your unfailing support made me who I am.

To patients from coastal South Carolina to foggy Northern California,
thank you. Your stories gifted this book life and light the way for others.

Finally, to my sweet boy Ben. Someday, we'll talk about
so much in heaven. Maybe even esophagus attacks.

CONTENTS

FOREWORD

I have known Dr. Doug Lake and his family for almost twenty years. A true joy of my nearly fifty years in academic radiology has been taking part in the education of students and residents, and I'm honored to have played a part in shaping the doctor Doug is today. He and I are both radiologists who regularly perform esophagograms on patients with reflux—and also good friends.

All of which is to say, I thought I knew Doug pretty well—until I read his book. As I read, I was surprised to learn about Doug's esophagus issues. I myself have chronic reflux disease—something I'd never shared with Doug.

This says a lot about the frequency of swallowing problems in the modern world.

And about how common it is for people to have chronic

reflux disease, and for that fact to remain unknown to even their families and close friends.

This book is a boon for anyone who experiences esophagus attacks. It explains often-confusing medical terminology in easily understood language, and simply and clearly describes symptoms, methods of diagnosis, and treatments. Best of all, Doug gives the reader simple and easy-to-follow steps to avoid developing acute symptoms and staying out of the emergency room, along with a great everyday approach to eating that can prevent attacks from ever starting.

Like Doug and his patients, over the years, I have learned things that control my own symptoms. But almost everyone will, like me, learn many new ways to make their lives better. And how great to not have to rely on trial and error to arrive at the best strategies!

This book will help the millions suffering from reflux and its complications. So, in addition to my congratulations to Doug, I would like to add my thanks—on behalf of all my patients, as well as myself.

STEPHEN I. SCHABEL, MD, FACR, FCCP
DISTINGUISHED UNIVERSITY PROFESSOR RADIOLOGY
MEDICAL UNIVERSITY OF SOUTH CAROLINA
CHARLESTON, SC

CHAPTER 1

ESOPHAGUS ATTACK? WHY DO I CARE?

Waves of severe chest pain.

Squeezing pain in the middle of my chest lasting three to six seconds.

Is this a heart attack? Should I call 911? Am I going to die?

But no pain radiating into my left arm, or my jaw, though I feel it in my lower neck, for sure.

Tension fills my shoulders, and I wipe my clammy hands on the napkin in my lap. I've never had pain like this before. Is there aspirin around?

Another wave of tearing pain hits my chest. I hunch forward slightly in my chair, and my legs push me back from the table. Deep exhale.

No, really, am I dying?

Stop. I ran a 5K in nineteen minutes this morning, and I'm a twenty-six-year-old medical student. This can't be a heart attack.

Then what the hell causes waves of chest pain? Why do I feel like someone grabbed a lemon squeezer from the kitchen and squeezed the middle of my chest?

Aortic dissection? Is my aorta rupturing in my chest?

Stop. It happened right after I ate that piece of the turkey thigh. It must be that. I hope it is that. Could food stuck in my esophagus feel like a vise gripping my chest?

Is this reflux?

No way. I've only eaten a protein bar and Gatorade, and that was after the 5K, almost six hours ago. I'm starving—I could eat a horse. There's nothing in my stomach. It's not reflux.

What is this?

Oh, no—does cancer do this?

What if this is cancer?

I had my first esophagus attack eighteen years ago when I was a third-year medical student. Even with my medical training, I was unable to identify, much less solve the problem of having food stuck in my esophagus. Since then, I have studied this problem extensively, from both a personal and a professional perspective. I have diagnosed and supported thousands of patients with this dilemma.

Experiencing esophagus attacks—the way I think of them when they happen to me, if not when I'm in my doctor role—are not only physically painful but also come with a significant emotional load as well. You must eat to live. If you can't eat food, you slowly die. Doctors can put tubes into parts of your body to help. Some need this, but the natural process of chewing and swallowing food is best. Eating represents a critical social gathering point around the world. Learning my steps to eating more comfortably and confidently solves the problem for most people. (Though if food does get stuck, you must see a medical professional).

This book will help you understand this problem and overcome it. You will learn about the esophagus. You will know you need to tell someone in the medical field about this problem. I will teach an easy 3-step process to help you eat more safely and confidently. I'll write about my approach to getting food unstuck and help you decide if you need to go to the emergency room. You will learn about other esophagus problems where the 3-step process helps.

In my own life, I eventually sought medical help, but I put it off longer than you might think. Perhaps the best part about swallowing—ha!—my pride and consulting a colleague was being able to put the worst fears out of my mind. No, this wasn't about my heart. No, I wasn't going to choke. No, this wasn't cancer.

Getting some basic answers from an expert lowered my stress level and allowed me to focus on doing what I could to understand and manage the way my body was working (and sometimes, not working so well).

My experience of how much fear esophagus attacks can instill is why I put so much emphasis in this book on addressing the many concerns, questions, and fears patients have brought me over the years. The list of fears can be long. It often includes:

Am I alone with this problem? No! Over 65,000 patients go to emergency rooms yearly in the US with food stuck in their esophagus. About 250,000 patients deal with problems with food impactions they can clear on their own each year in the US. Millions of Americans deal with gastroesophageal reflux disease (GERD), which we'll explain in later chapters and, when inadequately managed, likely contributes to this problem.

Do kids or young adults get this problem? Rarely. Food gets stuck for kids, and they can have pain while eating, but my solution doesn't apply to kids. I intend it only for adults. If you think food gets stuck for your child, please take them to their pediatrician, who may refer them to a pediatric gastroenterologist.

I'm so embarrassed about eating dinners with family or eating out with friends! I was, too! Steak houses used to be the worst for me. I'll teach you the strategy I have used to eat with confidence and overcome this fear.

I'm afraid of going to the emergency room to get food removed. That used to be me, too. Just the thought of a gigantic emergency room and surprise emergency endoscopy bills terrifies many patients. And they are right about this part: healthcare fails to provide price transparency. Most patients cannot guess their out-of-pocket cost. I don't have a clue, and I work in healthcare! In this book, you will learn how to discuss this with your healthcare provider and make a plan to avoid the emergency department and surprise medical bills.

What if I occasionally reflux? Can it progress to a bigger problem? We'll discuss reflux and the nonmedical and medical solutions. Knowledge will reduce anxiety. When you understand the problem, you own your answer.

Does a heart attack cause pain after swallowing food?

Usually no. For men, heart attacks have more typical presentations than this and often involve exertion. Women can have less obvious heart attack presentations. In chapter 3, you'll learn about what to expect during the workup of chest pain during eating.

Is this esophageal cancer? For 99 percent of you, no. For 1 percent, unfortunately, yes. I cannot teach you how to spot the difference. Your doctor cannot tell without testing. You must see a medical professional, and you'll read about that in chapter 3.

Where does it hurt? Point to your chest, to the fleshy part right above the breastbone in the midline, which doctors call the sternum. If you look at this book's front cover, it is the top of the lightning bolt. If your pain is at this spot, or below it to where the chest ends at the abdomen, immediately after you eat, this is what I'm calling an "esophagus attack," and this book is for to you.

This book does not help if your bowel is blocked. It is also not about choking or food going down the windpipe, known as the trachea. Choking on food in your windpipe is a different problem. If you are choking on food in your trachea, you need the Heimlich maneuver. You will suffocate and die if food sticks in your windpipe for more than a couple minutes. You can still breathe when food sticks in your esophagus rather than your trachea. Many patients confuse the two, so in this book, I'll explain how these differ.

This is not a diet book. This book teaches safe eating habits—eating healthfully is about avoiding food blockages rather than which calories or macronutrients you need.

This book emerges from my own pain and fear, as well as eighteen years of learning about and helping people with this problem.

Why learn from me? I'm the rare physician who has studied and treated a condition for eighteen years—and has it. I've helped thousands of patients. It's possible some others may know more than I do—I'm always learning. But I struggle with a problem you battle. I've had my own esophagus attacks. I want to help you manage, and even better, avoid them.

I am a diagnostic radiologist. This means I interpret medical imaging and perform image-guided procedures. In one typical scenario, I give patients a contrast called barium and take pictures of their esophagus. I help other doctors sort out their patients' esophagus problems. In my career, I've done thousands of these exams.

I developed my 3-step process to eat more easily for myself as well as my patients. As I began sharing with patients, it wasn't long before someone asked, "Will you write that down?" After that happened enough times, I searched Amazon to find a book to refer my patients to—and found nothing. So I bought *The Esophagus*, the esophagus medical bible. Eight hundred and thirteen pages dedicated to the esophagus. That must have chapters devoted to this problem and how to fix it, right? Well, esophageal strictures represent six pages of the book, mostly dedicated to pills, scopes, cameras, and balloons. Nothing addressed to the patient or what they can do.

Does this matter? Is food getting stuck in the esophagus a problem? Should I worry about my esophagus attacks? Remember the movie *Rocky*? Remember the song "The Eye of the Tiger?" Cue that song up in your head while you read the next paragraph.

You may battle fear, pain, self-loathing, shame, anxiety, and even depression from this problem. I've felt it and seen it. This is a genuine problem. You must work through emotional pain from this problem—they are your rivals.

If you're holding this book and food gets stuck, you're not alone. You hold a guide to work through this and emerge more confident that you can eat without pain or panic. You will understand how physicians test this problem and feel ready to speak with your own doctor. You will have a simple, 3-step method to eat more confidently and comfortably. You will eat out with your family and friends and know you can rely on this safe approach.

Step out of your fear cave. Want to embark on a journey to improve eating and stamp out fear? You must learn more! Let's go to Dr. Lake's version of medical school for the esophagus!

PART 1

WHAT'S GOING ON?

CHAPTER 2

MEDICAL SCHOOL FOR THE ESOPHAGUS

ANATOMY

"I've got that awful taste in my mouth again—like sucking on a sour grape. And that burning-embers sensation in my chest. Honey, would you mind finding my body pillow for me?"

Lauren struggles a bit to sit up in bed as her husband goes off in search of the requested item. Thirty-two weeks pregnant, she knows by now that the discomfort is connected to lying down. Maybe its pregnancy heartburn again, she thinks, though it didn't hurt like this last time. And there definitely wasn't the horrible-smelling breath before!

Lauren keeps swallowing saliva in hopes that will help. And she cycles through all her worries about what this could be. "My sinuses? They've been stuffed like a Build-a-Bear for months—thanks, pregnancy. The postnasal drip is driving me crazy—is it also causing this pain? Or maybe it has something to do with the baby weight I never got completely rid of after each of her first two? And what can I do about that anyway—like I have time to exercise! Maybe I have asthma. Could that make me feel like this? What if it's a heart problem?

"And how on earth am I ever going to get any sleep like this?"

Lauren's story is pretty typical. And answers aren't easy to get, especially because symptoms can be confused for signs of other conditions. Lauren, for example, is right that gastroesophageal reflux disease (GERD) is common in pregnancy. But it wasn't her whole story. (Fortunately, it turned out she had no reason to worry about her heart or her lungs.)

This chapter is my version of medical school but limited to consideration of the esophagus. In the process of becoming a doctor, medical school is when you get the basic science knowledge you'll need to care for patients—a key portion of that being anatomy. So that's where this chapter starts, with the anatomy—structure and function—of the esophagus and stomach. It includes a look at how they work together and at the critical process of swallowing food. This chapter lays the groundwork you need to understand what's going on in your body and in this book. It's the basic knowledge you'll need to take care of just one patient: you!

As a bonus, learning the facts is the best way to push away fears.

Admittedly, this is a lot of dry information, so I hope you'll bear with me while I help you get your bearings. If you want to skip ahead to the "what to do" chapters, I won't blame you for peeking ahead. But to get the best grounding for understanding your body, I hope you will return here to get a good grasp on the basics of how your esophagus works, and what can knock it off its game.

ANATOMY OVERVIEW

The esophagus is a muscular tube that connects your throat (pharynx) to your stomach. It is around twenty-three centimeters (nine inches) in length.

Your stomach is a sac-like structure located below your diaphragm.

The diaphragm is several muscles that divide the chest cavity from the abdominal cavity.

The chest cavity above the diaphragm muscle contains your heart, your lungs, your windpipe (trachea), and your esophagus. Your abdominal cavity below the diaphragm includes your stomach and the rest of your bowel, the liver, spleen, kidneys, and a bunch of other organs.

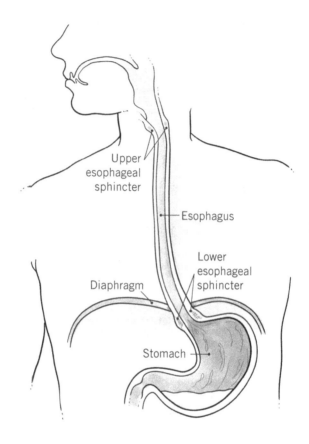

Upper esophageal sphincter

Esophagus

Lower esophageal sphincter

Diaphragm

Stomach

SPHINCTERS

You have strong muscles at the top and bottom of your esophagus—the upper and lower esophagus sphincters—that keep it closed most of the time. Your esophagus sphincters squeeze closed until you swallow. Swallowing opens these valves briefly, and then they close again.

You can think of these muscles a little like one-way valves. Your esophagus is like a garden hose. Imagine squeezing a garden hose, and how the hose will narrow, and how a firm enough grip could block anything from getting through that part of the hose. This is what the sphincters can do.

Humans average six hundred swallows per day and fifty swallows overnight. When you swallow, you initiate a chain of events where sphincters open and close. Esophagus muscles contract and relax in wave-like patterns to push food along. When Lauren lies in bed and swallows, her saliva passes through the upper sphincter, then the lower sphincter, on the way to her stomach. As she swallows saliva, she flushes acid out of her esophagus. Swallowing saliva protects the esophagus and neutralizes acid.

LES

The lower esophageal sphincter (LES) is found where the esophagus meets the stomach, at the diaphragm. It is around three to four centimeters in length, so between 1.2 to 1.7 inches. Its job is to keep the "bottom" end of the esophagus closed, stopping reflux of anything from the stomach back into the esophagus.

This is where most patients I see get food stuck above the LES.

Since the LES occurs where the stomach, or as the doctors say "gastro," meets the esophagus, it is also called the gastro-esophageal junction (GEJ). Technically, the GEJ and LES are slightly different entities. For this book, you'll only have to worry about the LES. Hormones mess with the LES, so Lauren's pregnancy worsens her GERD.

UES

Your upper esophagus sphincter, at the "top" of the esophagus, is responsible for keeping the tube closed at that end until it is time to swallow. The dominant muscle in the UES is the one that prevents upward reflux from the esophagus to the trachea. It stops gastric contents from entering the lungs. If you think about the esophagus as a battlefield, the upper esophagus sphincter is the final line of defense against stomach acid entering the trachea (windpipe) and lungs.

You cannot directly control your esophagus sphincters. You indirectly control them by swallowing. Swallowing initiates complex nerve and chemical signals that cause your esophageal muscles and sphincters to allow food to pass. It is so complicated that experts don't fully understand it, so you don't need to either. Just know you do consciously control the initiation of swallowing.

STOMACH

Stomach cells secrete acid to break down food and start digestion. The acid your stomach uses is powerful. Your stomach handles the acid without a problem. The problems start if the acid gets out of the stomach and back into the esophagus.

Your GI tract is meant to be a one-way street. Food and acid move in their intended direction with no problem. Food moves from your mouth, down your esophagus, into your stomach, then into the small bowel and beyond. The stomach handles acid well. Your pancreas secretes neutralizing liquid in the next segment of your bowel after the stomach, the duodenum. This neutralizing fluid takes care of the acid. If the acid from the stomach enters the esophagus, we get reflux and problems—no neutralizing happens in that direction. For Lauren, the sour taste, foul smell, sinus pressure, and postnasal drip represent problems from reflux. Refluxed acid enters her sinuses, causing pressure and the postnasal drip. The sour taste and foul smell are also from refluxed acid.

ESOPHAGUS LINING

The cells on the inside of the esophagus are different from the cells of the stomach. They are not designed to contend with strong acid, which is fine, as long as the valves stay closed.

Stomach acid will damage the cells on the inside of the esophagus over time. More on this in chapter 12.

GER

Stomach acid entering the esophagus is reflux, specifically gastroesophageal reflux, which is abbreviated GER. Also known as uncomplicated reflux. If Lauren *only* had the funny taste in her mouth, she would simply have GER.

When, a few minutes later, Lauren developed pain with GER,

it became GERD, or gastroesophageal reflux disease, also known as esophagitis. Nonpainful reflux = GER. Painful reflux = GERD. In GERD, stomach acid irritates the esophagus, causing chest pain. Lauren's postnasal drip, sinus pressure, and asthma are more elusive hints of GERD.

GER happens occasionally to healthy people and is considered okay. As long as there is no pain, and no other issues, no problem.

GERD

GERD is the *painful* movement of material from the stomach up the esophagus. That's unpleasant in the moment but also puts you at risk for bigger problems. When GERD goes untreated for years or decades, the esophagus can be slowly damaged in ways that cause more serious issues later in life.

In GERD, usually the esophagus has been damaged by stomach acid, but other things like radiation therapy for esophageal cancer, chemotherapy, or an infection can also damage the esophagus.

You've scraped your knee before, right? The skin before the scrape is your usual shade of skin color. After the injury, you scraped a few skin layers off. It hurts, right? Stings! Maybe the skin turns pink or red. Exposing your esophagus to stomach acid injures your esophagus, like scraping your knee. A similar process of injury where the top layer or two of cells get injured. The esophagus even looks pink or red on the inside when it's injured. When the esophagus is irritated or injured, that's GERD.

Over long enough periods of time, untreated GERD damages the esophagus. Chronic acid exposure in the esophagus signals to esophagus cells (which don't like acid) to change to stomach cells (which don't mind it). Even the experts aren't sure how this happens, but they agree it isn't good. Many think the change in cells may worsen reflux because it results in the esophagus not closing as effectively. Other cells in our immune system rush in to help but may be part of the problem. More on that in chapter 12.

If GERD continues, two different things can happen. One, the esophagus can narrow, which is called an esophageal stricture. This stricture or narrowing is where food gets stuck. Two, as the cells change from healthy esophagus cells to stomach cells, they can be injured in ways that break the cell DNA and proteins. This kind of damage can result in esophageal cancer. This is rare, and again experts aren't sure of the exact mechanism behind this change to cancer, but we know it happens.

Lauren was experiencing GERD because she was pregnant and had a chocolate mint milkshake an hour before bedtime. Some stomach acid moved up into her esophagus, and the result was very unpleasant. Hormones related to pregnancy relax the lower esophagus sphincter and contribute to reflux. The pressure of the baby may also have contributed. If you have GERD during pregnancy, you must bring it up to your healthcare provider. So, Lauren needed symptom relief in the moment, and a plan to make sure symptoms couldn't go on long enough to cause lasting damage. And she needed to get to the bottom of it so she wouldn't go on stressing herself by imagining terrible things her symptoms might mean.

HIATAL HERNIA

A hiatal hernia is another common problem of the distal esophagus that contributes to GERD. You've probably heard of a hernia. A hernia occurs when some part of your body squeezes through an opening it shouldn't. The hernia that happens at the junction of the esophagus and the stomach is called a hiatal hernia. When this happens, part of the stomach slides up into the chest. No one is 100 percent sure how this happens. Still, the widening of the opening in the diaphragm and loss of the connective tissues surrounding the LES probably contribute most. Overeating is the biggest source of blame for hiatal hernias. Physicians guess that when the stomach stretches, it tugs at the esophagus a little and weakens the connections between the lower esophagus and the diaphragm. Maybe the diaphragm is stretched wider at the same time? No one is sure, but we know hiatal hernias develop and enlarge.

DIAPHRAGM

A hiatal hernia contributes to GERD because the LES shifts upward above the diaphragm. The diaphragm reinforces the muscles of the LES, allowing those muscles to close better. If the lower sphincter is an inch (2.5 centimeters) above the diaphragm, the lower sphincter loses its strengthening buddy. I think about two people who bear hug each other to illustrate how the LES and diaphragm work together. First, hug yourself. In other words, cross your arms in front of yourself, so your right hand touches your left upper arm, and your left hand touches your right upper arm. Your forearms probably touch your chest. The space between your arms and your chest is the esophagus. Your arms are the muscle surrounding the distal esophagus. Now, imagine a second person walking up behind you, wrapping their arms over yours and bear-hugging you. The second person is the diaphragm wrapping around the LES. Together, these two sets of arms squeeze the esophagus closed.

Now, take the bear-hug arms and shift them to your waist. The two sets of arms don't overlap anymore, and neither is as strong as they were together. When a hiatal hernia develops, the diaphragm doesn't surround the esophageal sphincter. Separated, both are weaker. The esophagus doesn't close well, and gastric acid moves up to the esophagus, i.e., GER. Later in chapter 12, we'll discuss surgeries to fix hiatal hernias and repair the diaphragm.

ESOPHAGUS MUSCLES

Your esophagus is mostly muscle. The upper third of your esophagus muscles are striated muscle, like the muscles you exercise at a gym. The lower two-thirds of the esophagus is smooth muscle. Smooth muscle contracts and relaxes in waves. Esophagus contraction waves move food toward your stomach about 2.5–5 centimeters per second. In other words, your food moves one to two inches downward per second as your esophagus contracts and pushes it downward. A normal contraction wave typically lasts about seven seconds. The esophagus muscle contracts so powerfully, the esophagus shortens 2–2.5 centimeters when it contracts. As you swallow, esophagus muscles contract to force food down, and the sphincters open to allow food into the stomach.

Q. Gastroesophageal Reflux Disease (GERD), if left untreated, over decades can:

1. Cause chronic pain after eating.

2. Slowly damage the esophagus and can cause a stricture.

3. Cause a premalignant condition called Barrett's esophagus but rarely cause esophageal cancer.

4. All of the above.

Answer: 4. All of the above.

The esophagus muscles and sphincters can reverse. Burping is the retrograde flow of gas from the stomach. Vomiting is the retrograde flow of stomach contents. Both are important when you need it.

When Lauren experienced reflux, she could taste the acid, and she was anxious about the whole thing. Does that happen for you? Perhaps after a big meal? It happens for me about once every two months. I used to worry about it. Please remember that reflux occurs from time to time in healthy people. If it doesn't cause pain or other problems, occasional reflux is normal. When reflux happens—even if there's no pain—I encourage you to drink water. Not Coke. Not Pepsi. Nothing with strong acid. Tap water is best. It will flush out acid and return the esophagus to a neutral nonacidic state and prevent damage. If you don't have tap water handy, swallow your saliva.

GEJ PRESSURE

Another design of the esophagus preventing reflux is its closed pressure of 20 mmHg. You've had your blood pressure taken before, right? Normal blood pressure is less than 120/80 mmHg. Anything over 140/90 is considered hypertension. LES pressure of 20 mmHg is sufficient to close the sphincter. The LES relaxes one to two-and-a-half seconds after you swallow to allow the food bolus to pass. Then the LES contracts again, and the closed resting pressure of 20 mmHg returns. Several factors alter how well the LES opens. The food bolus itself (solid, liquid, or combination), gravity, the pressure differences between the abdominal cavity and chest cavity, and the diaphragm position all affect LES opening. Taking in deep breaths contracts the diaphragm muscle and raises the sphincter pressure by up to 5 mmHg. A deep breath changes the position and angle of the LES. File this tidbit away because you will come back to breathing and diaphragm position when we try to get food "unstuck."

OGILVIE SCALE

OGILVIE NUMBER	LEVEL OF DIFFICULTY	SEE A DOCTOR?	WHEN TO SEE DOCTOR?
0	No problems at all.	No.	Not applicable.
1	Avoid certain foods.	Yes.	This month.
2	Semi-solid diet only.	Yes.	This week.
3	Fluids only.	Yes.	Today or next business day. Consider urgent care if available.
4	No fluids pass at all.	Yes.	Visit ER now.

The Ogilvie scale is the last thing to learn in medical school for the esophagus. There are five levels on the Ogilvie scale (0-4). The scale rates the level of difficulty swallowing (i.e., dysphagia) you have. Perfect is 0, and you have no problems swallowing anything. Ogilvie 1 is a regular diet avoiding certain foods (steak, chicken, bread, etc.). Ogilvie 2 is when only a semi-solid diet works. Ogilvie 3 is when only fluids will pass. Ogilvie 4 is complete dysphagia to even liquids. If you're a 1 or 2, you should make an appointment to see your doctor about this problem. If you're a 3, you should call your doctor immediately or on the next reasonable day to make an appointment. If you're a 4 on this scale, you should go to an emergency room now.

Lauren was an Ogilvie 0 patient with no problems swallowing except for pain. If Lauren doesn't treat her GERD, over time, she will accrue lasting damage to her esophagus. Chronic injury can slowly narrow the esophagus, which can lead to food getting stuck. In this case, Lauren may become an Ogilvie 1 or 2. I was an Ogilvie 1 when Thanksgiving turkey caused my first esophagus attack (chapter 1). If Lauren's GERD progressed in her thirties or forties, she might start avoiding the foods that get stuck, like steak or chicken. It might make her more apprehensive around mealtimes. Eating out with a social group might become a nightmare.

But let's say Lauren goes to her doctor to discuss her symptoms, gets treatment, heals her esophagus, and goes back to getting a good night's sleep even when she's enjoyed a milkshake. Details of this kind of esophagus treatment are coming up in the next chapter. GERD should not hold Lauren back from her life, cause pain, or prolong frustration.

Still, a patient like Lauren might still have worries. Can I afford this? What tests are appropriate? Will my doctor order the right ones? Do I take these medicines with pain or all the time? Can I take over the counter versions, or must I take the prescription ones?

Working through esophagus problems is only partly about the esophagus. It is also about years of uncertainty, pain, frustration, and anxiety. You can push back against all that by learning more. That's the project chapter 3 continues, with a look at what doctors do for esophagus problems.

CHAPTER 3

RESIDENCY FOR THE ESOPHAGUS

PRACTICAL APPLICATION

"Yeah, Doc, this does suck. You know what? 'Suck' really doesn't cover something this all-around awful. Some days, I don't want to get out of bed. The physical toll is one thing, and I'm adjusting. The emotional toll is the beast no one discusses. You think you have this great life planned, and then suddenly you're on this horror-movie detour, and there's no way back. My wife and kids look at me differently. Everything in medicine is so expensive. I'm not working, and insurance, even with disability insurance, only covers so much. There's so much unknown, sometimes even my doctors are just guessing. The only thing I know for sure is I don't want to die young like my dad."

Joe was in his late thirties when he began having problems

with food getting stuck. It went on for months, and only got worse, so eventually, he went to the doctor where he received a diagnosis of esophageal cancer. This is a disease that strikes at the median age of sixty-eight. (Remember, 99 percent of people experiencing esophagus attacks don't have cancer, but 1 percent do. In other words, there's a 99 percent chance something else is causing your esophagus attack.)

I met Joe after he'd had chemoradiation therapy but before surgery. His cancer was curable, but he faced a difficult road. The thoughts he shared with me clearly reflected that.

In someone under forty like Joe, esophageal cancer goes from a one-in-one-hundred thing to a one-in-*100,000* thing. So I'm not bringing him up here to scare you; in all likelihood, your symptoms have nothing to do with cancer. It's important to look at Joe's story, though, because it underlines a few things. 1) Cancer of the esophagus is rare, but I've heard many patients confess they dreaded it. So don't waste energy worrying until it is proven you should worry. 2) Fear of a disastrous diagnosis keeps a surprising number of people from seeking treatment. This, of course, is terribly counterproductive. Seek answers and relief! 3) Any issue with your health brings emotional baggage with it, and it is important to deal with that component of the situation, too. And finally, 4) Your symptoms *are* treatable, and way, way more easily than what Joe was enduring. Doctors *can* treat GERD, swallowing problems, and other symptoms. They can stop pain and heal the esophagus.

If chapter 2 was esophagus medical school, chapter 3 is esophagus residency. That's what doctors call the education and training after medical school. It's called residency because so much time is spent at the hospital, you almost live there. So we're getting a little more in-depth here and starting a more practical orientation to the material. You're not in a classroom or library anymore. You're in the hospital learning on the job from other doctors and from your experiences with real patients. A main focus here will be medical testing of esophagus problems.

Remember: knowledge is power. As you learn more, fear loosens its grip.

TAKE A BREATH

So much about health issues creates so much uncertainty and anxiety. Even just reading about it can stir up negative feelings. So I want you to practice a little calming maneuver right now if you feel it will be helpful. Even if you don't think you need it now, give it a try. Practice it from time to time. Then take it with you into your interactions with your esophagus and your medical care, drawing on it anytime you need to ease your tension.

Here it is: breathe. Take in a deep breath and let it out slowly.

More specifically, try a three-second breath in your nose and blow it out of your mouth over a four-count. Before you read or do anything else, complete that cycle eight more times.

911, WHAT'S YOUR EMERGENCY?

Patients enter the healthcare system with difficulty swallowing in two ways: through their regular doctor or through the emergency room.

Pro tip: Seeing your regular doctor outperforms the ER route for everything except an actual emergency. Seeing your regular doctor is the way to never get to that emergency state!

I'll get to the process with your regular doctor in the next chapter, but here we'll begin with what happens via an emergency room. Joe went directly to his doctor with his symptoms and avoided the ER. That is definitely preferable if it is possible.

So, you're at home, and food is stuck. You could try my approach from chapter 5: What to Do When Food Is Stuck. But please don't spend over five to ten minutes trying these tricks before seeking professional attention.

Then comes the point when you're finding someone to drive you to the nearest emergency room or calling 911.

Let's say you call 911.

"911; what's your emergency?"

"I am having pain in my chest after I ate. I think it has to do with eating, but it might be a heart attack."

They'll ask you to describe the pain you're feeling. For me, pain arrives in waves when food is stuck. It's worst immediately after I've swallowed something that got stuck. I sip liquid when something is stuck. No solid food during an esophagus attack. Each sip of liquid unleashes new waves of squeezing pain (more on this in chapter 5).

If your description involves chest pain, just know a paramedic will think about heart problems first. They will slap EKG leads on your chest, shove an oxygen tube in your nose and give you an aspirin to swallow. You'll get strapped to a stretcher, an IV will be started in your arm, and you'll be rushed to the nearest hospital. Please don't be anxious. It's brand new for you, but paramedics care for people quickly all the time. They're doing their job the right way, even if your problem turns out to have nothing to do with your heart.

EMERGENCY ROOM

Once you get to the emergency room, there will be a variety of ways an ER will handle you. You'll likely be transported to a room, and a nurse or two will introduce themselves. If you don't have an IV yet, expect one. Lab tests will be drawn from the IV, including labs for a heart attack.

So there's a lot going on in the emergency room, and it can be overwhelming. But it is all to help you, remember. Don't let it provoke anxiety. You should also know there are around 62,500 emergency room visits yearly in the U.S. for food getting stuck in the esophagus. Esophagus attacks are frequent. ER's are familiar with this. You are in experienced hands.

ER DOCTOR

An emergency room physician or physician assistant will see you. They'll ask you to re-explain what caused you to call 911. They will order the tests you need and may be the one to tell you the results of those tests. These tests are described below. Also below is information on the medications ER doctors may prescribe. In the ER, doctors may also order procedures or call on doctors from other specialties to evaluate and help you. Depending upon their level of concern about a heart problem, an ER doctor may admit you to the hospital.

CHEST X-RAY

You will likely have a chest X-ray. The ER doctor and radiology doctor (i.e., radiologist) look carefully to see if your esophagus ruptured. They look for gas in the middle of your chest or gas in your upper abdomen. Your doctors look for other severe problems like you swallowed a non-food object like metal. Children are notorious for eating coins.

Swallowed chicken or fish bones are common but may be challenging to see on X-rays. Finally, swallowed batteries are a medical emergency. The coin-shaped lithium batteries found in watches are horrible. They discharge electricity in the esophagus, make a hole, and cause severe damage. A gastroenterologist, otolaryngologist, or general surgeon will need to remove a button battery with an endoscope, which is covered in more detail later in this chapter.

CT SCAN

You may undergo computed tomography (i.e., CT or CAT scan). The CT machine looks like a big donut: it is a large circle with a hole in the middle.

The machine sends X-rays through you and detects which parts of your body block them to create images. The radiologist looks at your images and searches for problems from impacted food. They search for a hole (i.e., perforation) or infection (i.e., mediastinitis, abscess formation, or enteric fistula). Usually, we infuse a fluid called contrast in your IV. Contrast contains iodine and helps radiologists see blood vessels and structures with blood flow, including your esophagus.

I know all this sounds scary, but I invite you to step out of the fear cave. I've been looking at CTs for years, and I have seen two real-life examples of esophageal rupture from food impaction. But only two. I've read five to ten CT exams of the chest a day, five days a week, for at least the last eleven years, since my actual residency ended. That's over 10,000 CT exams of the chest, and I've seen two food bolus impactions cause an esophageal rupture. It happens, but it's rare. So try to keep in mind that the doctors have to check. If this is your problem, you definitely cannot let it go undetected, but it is highly unlikely this is what is happening. By the time I met Joe, he had undergone several CT exams, and they no longer provoked anxiety.

ESOPHAGRAM

Doctors ask radiologists to find out if there is a hole or rupture of the esophagus. Sometimes, radiologists ask you to drink a liquid ("contrast") that tastes like a chalky milkshake, while they take pictures. However, the liquid you drink for the exam can make it harder for the doctor who puts the scope and camera down your esophagus to see things. The CT exam is superior to look for esophagus rupture. I saw Joe for his second esophagram and fortunately, there was no sign his cancer was back. Unfortunately, radiation treatment had caused new swallowing problems. More on this in chapter 12.

ER MEDS

Doctors may try to help the food pass through your esophagus by giving you different medicines. If medications help while you're in the ER, that's fantastic! You avoid an invasive procedure!

Helpful medicines either relax your esophagus muscles, produce gas, or do both. Emergency room doctors give "cocktails" of several drugs together. You might drink sodium bicarbonate, simethicone, citric acid, and water together. At the same time, a nurse might give you 0.5-1.0 mg glucagon into your IV. This combination therapy does four things to help food through a blockage. Glucagon relaxes the esophagus muscles. The esophagus clamps down on food that's stuck, and making the muscle relax helps. Sometimes, glucagon works by itself. The effervescent agent forms gas in your esophagus, similar to but much more than Pepsi or Coke do. It combines one teaspoon of sodium bicarbonate and citric acid with 30 mL of water to produce 400 mL of CO_2. A twelve-ounce can of Coke is around 330 mL of liquid. In other words, a teaspoon of effervescent agent makes more gas in your esophagus than there is liquid in a can of Coke! The water generates hydrostatic pressure to help food pass. In other words, the weight of the water pushes impacted food down. You get the cocktail sitting up, and gravity helps food pass. Gas and water create pressure on your lower esophageal sphincter while glucagon relaxes your sphincter. The impacted food, hopefully, slides into your stomach. With these medicines, doctors helped food pass in twelve out of sixteen patients in a small trial published in the *American Journal of Roentgenology* in 1990—a 75 percent success rate.

Another study used one or two agents rather than four to see if it worked as well. Gas-making effervescent agents alone helped 55.6 percent of patients pass the food obstruction. Glucagon by itself succeeded for almost 18 percent of patients. In another trial of 645 patients in Minnesota, 36.8 percent of food impactions passed with glucagon only, as reported in the *United European Gastroenterology Journal* in 2019.

INGREDIENT	ROUTE	FUNCTION
SODIUM BICARBONATE	By mouth	Combines with #2 to produce gas.
CITRIC ACID	By mouth	Combines with #1 to produce gas.
SIMETHICONE	By mouth	Helps relieve pain from gas.
WATER	By mouth	Lubrication and minimal pressure.
GLUCAGON	IV	Relaxes esophagus muscle.

(Don't worry too much about those who didn't respond to the drugs, by the way. They all went on to have a scope put into their esophagus, and 100 percent of those patients passed the blocked food successfully that way.)

OTHER MEDICATIONS

I want to mention three other medications, even though they aren't generally as successful, because they may come up. Benzodiazepine medications, most commonly Diazepam at 2.5-10 mg through your IV, rarely helps but might be tried. Diazepam, or Valium, helps you relax, which should help your esophagus relax. Calcium channel blockers relax the esophagus but not as well as glucagon. Oral nitroglycerin, usually given during a heart attack, may relax the esophagus.

Notice a common theme—relax the esophagus muscle? We'll return to this idea in chapter 5.

AVOID PAPAIN

Papain tenderizes meat with enzymes. This meat tenderizer is also a medicine given in the emergency room to help if food is stuck. It breaks down beef, chicken, pork, etc. If beef gets stuck, a chemical that breaks down meat might help, right? What could go wrong? Your esophagus is muscle. Meat is muscle. In a few extreme cases where patients swallowed papain in the emergency room, as directed by a doctor, the papain ate through the esophagus, created a hole, and patients died from later complications. No papain!

This book empowers you to know what to expect—and what to refuse—when it comes to your healthcare. Advocate against papain for your safety.

SPECIALISTS

Emergency room staff treat on their own, but they may also ask for advice and help: a "consult" from another physician in a different medical specialty.

ER doctors often ask for help from doctors skilled at advancing a scope to fix food blockages. At most hospitals, the ER doctor consults a gastroenterologist who helps the patient. Sometimes, an otolaryngologist (i.e., ENT or ear, nose, and throat doctor), a surgeon, or a family medicine doctor may help. Joe met a gastroenterologist (GI doctor). Joe's GI doctor became a key member of his care team and critical to helping him navigate new challenges.

So if medications don't help and the consulting physician arrives to help you pass the obstructed food, what will you experience?

ENDOSCOPY LAB

You'll travel on a gurney or wheelchair from the ER to the endoscopy center. You will enter a holding area before the endoscopy room. Your ER nurse may help the endoscopy doctor (GI, ENT, surgeon, etc.). Usually, you will meet a new nurse. Your nurse explains the procedure and what to expect afterward. You will meet the doctor here or as you enter the endoscopy room. They also explain the procedure, risks, benefits, and alternatives. You will sign a document granting their permission to help you, also known as consent. All this can be intimidating, but my patient Joe has had several endoscopy procedures, and he'd tell you they're mostly a breeze.

The endoscopy nurse or staff will take you into the endoscopy room. Usually, you will lie on your right side. You should have a plastic tube called a nasal cannula giving you oxygen in your nose. They will perform a time-out procedure. Medical time-outs are critical safety checks ensuring the right procedure on the right patient for the right reason is being done. At this point, the endoscopy nurse will give you medications in your IV, most commonly versed and fentanyl. Propofol is an option, but an anesthesiologist is usually required, and that costs more. Most patients don't remember anything from this point until afterward.

The endoscopy doctor safely advances the scope. It is best to imagine a thin garden hose about 9 mm in diameter, so about 0.38 inch. The scope is a little bigger than a McDonald's straw (7.2 mm or 0.28 inch in diameter). Pencils are 5 mm in diameter, so two pencils next to one another is a little bigger than the scope. The doctor advances a flexible scope down your esophagus. They take pictures along the way.

They have two options for your food blockage. Gently pushing the food through the sphincter is option one. In option two, piecemeal removal takes a little food out at a time. Gentle pushing used to be frowned upon as recently as 2011, but new guidelines say gentle pushing is safe. Three hundred and seventy-five patients in two recent studies had the gentle pushing approach without esophageal perforation. And removing food in bits requires a lot more time.

Because you presented with food impaction, your doctor must consider eosinophilic esophagitis (EoE). EoE was rare thirty years ago but is a common cause of food impactions today. What might you need to know about EoE while in the ER? Your doctor should biopsy your esophagus when they clear your food impaction. Bleeding, esophagus tear, or another problem are all reasons to skip the biopsy. But, if they can, they should take cells from the esophagus and look for EoE. You'll learn more about EoE in chapter 12.

You may need to advocate for yourself about this. If you can't, bring your pushy sister or bossy aunt and ask them to be your advocate. If your esophagus is entirely normal, it is essential to perform the biopsy. This sounds counterintuitive, right? What doctor in their right mind sticks a needle into a normal esophagus? An EoE esophagus commonly looks normal. So, advocate for a biopsy.

You should know, even with all this, there is a silver lining. Esophagus attack, 911, rushed to the hospital, ER bill—what could possibly be the silver lining?

It's this: you (usually) meet a gastroenterologist.

That person or one of their partners helps you throughout this process. You'll learn more about their role in chapter 4, but for now, appreciate the fact that they meet you at your worst point with impacted food, and that allows them to take that experience and knowledge of your situation into the longer-term project of caring for you.

BACK AT HOME

Once the food impaction is cleared—either with medications in the ER or in the endoscopy suite—expect to go home. Unless there is a complication, there is no need to keep you in the hospital. If your pain resolves, further heart tests make no sense. Most ER doctors test for an elevated troponin level to screen for a heart attack. If the level is normal, you're not having a heart attack. The GI doctor who cleared the blocked food will make an appointment with you for follow-up. Or the ER doctor will refer you to another gastroenterologist or back to your primary care doctor. Each hospital system handles these details differently.

Getting you to see the best doctor to fix your esophagus is the ultimate goal. Fixing the blocked food helps, definitely, but it is only the first step.

My patient Joe had been through many of these medical interventions at one time or another on his way to his diagnosis. Tough as some of them can be, the relief they can bring usually makes it worthwhile, even for Joe, where there were no easy answers. Because he sought help without delay, doctors found his cancer early, meaning the best treatments were given the best chance of working effectively.

Encountering Joe as a patient shook me to my core. I think because he could have been me. Except Joe was a better man than me because he did not hesitate to take his symptoms to his doctor. I hid in my fear for years, all the issues around food getting stuck, the anxiety, the uncertainty.

Fortunately for me, my journey through the medical system *as a patient* followed a much more typical course, once I finally sought help. The majority of my care has taken place in outpatient settings, rather than the ER, and that's what I recommend to anyone, to the degree it's possible to control it. The next chapter follows that doctor's-office course, to show you what you can expect—and benefit from—when dealing with food blockages of the esophagus.

CHAPTER 4

FELLOWSHIP FOR THE ESOPHAGUS

SPECIALIZATION

"I feel relief after telling you all this, doctor. I wasn't sure I needed to see a specialist or anyone, but I keep having this trouble swallowing, and it's frustrating, as well as painful. And I was feeling so uncertain about what it is and what to do. But using only 'Dr. Google' was only making it worse. I was so anxious about what might be found if I saw a doctor!"

Phyllis had a decades-long relationship with her primary care physician, whom she thoroughly trusted. But still, she waited to bring up her trouble swallowing until she started to feel really desperate. Ultimately, the relief she found began simply with sharing her problem with an expert. But on her first visit to the office, her worries were evident as she described her problem: pain in her chest after she ate, mostly with meat and bread.

Phyllis' experience in the gastroenterologist's office is typical of the kind of medical care this chapter is about. We're moving out of the emergency room now—always better to avoid emergencies than to treat them—and into your regular doctor's office. We'll look at what you can expect as your doctor evaluates your difficulty swallowing, or "dysphagia."

This is what I'm calling the fellowship part of your esophagus medical training. After residency, many physicians go right into practice. But some continue for more training in a specialty or subspecialty, making a huge step up in patient responsibility at the same time. This chapter moves away from emergency removal of food obstruction to outpatient evaluation and treatment, often under the care of one of these specialists. Your knowledge base is about to get more in-depth, too.

It was with a fellowship-trained gastroenterologist that Phyllis consulted about her swallowing problems. She explained that for about a month, she'd experienced pain right where her neck meets her chest, which happened right after she ate. It felt like the food just didn't want to go down. She described the feeling of something squeezing in her chest, on and off for five or ten seconds at a time. Squeeze, release, squeeze, release.

Answering her doctor's questions, she filled in more details. No symptoms with exercise. Sometimes, the pain in her lower neck extended more into her chest, but never into her jaw or down her arm. No change in breathing, no coughing. As Phyllis explained, she started to swallow fine, but then it feels like the food just gets stuck. No trouble chewing, no mouth pain. No smoking, no more than a glass or two of wine in a week. It never happens with liquids, just solid food.

The doctor's questions eliminate heart problems and choking. Orders for lab tests and a swallowing study with a radiologist are sent in, and the results of those will determine what, if anything, else needs to be done. Phyllis schedules a follow-up appointment for two weeks later. As the doctor explained, Phyllis was wise to come in before this became an emergency and she ended up in the ER.

The doctor also asked about and listened to Phyllis' concerns and fears and addressed them. Most of all, pointing out that all her feelings around the subject were normal, and that taking a positive step to deal with her health and safety was in itself important, and showed a commitment to her own well-being.

All in all, it was a typical encounter for difficult swallowing. Your meeting with a primary care provider or specialist might sound like this, or it might be different. Each patient and physician have a unique relationship, unique goals of care, and unique priorities. Medical practice elegantly blends science and art to help each patient. But there will be common elements to the workup for swallowing problems, and that's what this chapter explains in greater detail.

For a person who experiences food getting stuck from time to time, even if you get it unstuck on your own, it's a good idea to tell your healthcare provider. In fact, you need to do this. I cannot overstate this. Remember the 99/1 rule? Ninety-nine of one hundred will NOT have cancer, but one will. Liberate your mind from cancer fear and make that appointment! Tell them up front swallowing food is hard.

Like Phyllis, you'll experience relief after discussing your issue with a doctor. You may find an emotional weight lifts from your shoulders, just as Phyllis felt her anxiety and uncertainty evaporate once she saw there was someone who could help her get this under control. Phyllis would be the first one to tell you: go get your question checked out.

ASKED AND ANSWERED

When I finally got it together to go see a doctor myself, I waded through all these same questions. I experienced from the other side what it's like to answer rather than ask these questions.

Physicians ask open-ended questions and let the patient talk.

Tell them your story, unfiltered. If you're not sure where to start or what's essential, below are standard questions. The answers in italics are my own. My answers are not yours; I'm merely giving you my answers as an example of the kind of details I needed to share.

What happens to cause this?

It happens when I swallow solid food, mostly beef, chicken, or pork, but it occurs with sushi and bread. It happens anytime I eat too quickly or eat without liquid.

When does it happen?

I can feel it come on within five seconds of swallowing if I will have a problem.

Describe the pain.

Two- to five-second waves of grabbing pain occur in my chest. If the piece of food is small or barely blocking, the pain is mild. Maybe a three or four out of ten. Imagine squeezing a therapy ball...that squeezing pain. Other times, I describe the sensation as a fullness or pressure in the middle of my chest. If a big chunk blocks my esophagus, the squeezing pain worsens. Say a seven or eight out of ten pain. It doesn't have a stabbing or piercing quality. Remember when I broke my wrist, and Dr. Friederich opened it up and fixed it? When the nerve block wore off, I had ten out of ten stabbing, piercing pain. Blocked food pain never approaches broken bone pain.

How long does the pain last?

At first, I get waves of pain, lasting thirty to sixty seconds. If I don't drink any liquid, the vise-like squeezing fades to a sense of fullness in the middle of my chest. After another sip of water, the encircling squeezing waves of pain return. I never eat more solid food if something is stuck. It never helps. The intensity ratchets up another point or two on the scale if I eat solid food.

What have you tried to help this?

Laughing out loud You have no idea how many different things I've tried! Look at my smile—this book distills eighteen years of patient encounters and personal experiments into a how-to guide. I ask every patient what makes it better for them. Everything that works for others and me ends up here.

What makes this worse?

More solid food never works. Hoping this goes away on its own doesn't work. Ignoring my uncertainty, fears, and frustration walked me down a dark stairway to an emotional basement where I didn't tell my wife or friends. Storing these emotions in the far corner of my emotional basement ate at me until I faced the problem. I sat with it, told my wife, got help, and wrote a book.

How long has this been going on? Days, weeks, months, years, decades?

Eighteen years, give or take.

Tell me more about how this makes you feel. (This one wasn't part of my own training but is critical for the patient to tell the physician, because it further humanizes the problem.)

The first time this happened, I was scared. So, so scared. I moved through heart attack, aortic dissection, and GERD, but my mind latched onto, "What if it's cancer?" I was worried about what my family would think. I didn't tell anyone for years. I shrunk up into my fear basement.

So just do it. Make an appointment. Sit with your fears and write them down.

Think about answers to those questions.

Consider journaling about food getting stuck.

But whatever else you do, *see your healthcare provider.*

WHO TO TELL?

Patients ask me who to tell. Telling SOMEONE is the hardest step. I'm not limiting. Tell your primary care physician (i.e., PCP). They are the best. For most, that will be a family medicine physician, internal medicine physician, or obstetrics and gynecology physician. Phyllis told her family medicine physician. Tell a medical doctor or a doctor of osteopathy (i.e., DO).

You may receive healthcare from a mid-level provider such as a nurse practitioner (NP), a physician assistant (i.e., PA), or an advanced practice registered nurse (APRN). If so, tell them!

If you are seeing a speech therapist already for another issue, tell them! They will probably say, "Tell your primary doctor." But they will positively encourage you to tell your doctor.

Tell your dentist! Your dentist focuses on your teeth, and they will say to tell your doctor, but chewing food with good teeth helps people who struggle with food sticking.

What about a chiropractor? They will say, "Tell your primary doctor." Expert physicians don't fully understand the relationship of the vagus nerve, thoracic spinal nerves, and the esophagus. If you see a chiropractor, tell them and your primary doctor.

If you are seeing a therapist or psychiatrist, they also fall into the category of needing to know you're having this problem.

They will help you, but they will encourage you to see your primary doctor.

Are you already seeing a gastroenterologist (GI doctor), for something else? Boom! Perfect! Tell them.

If you're seeing another medical specialist, tell them and ask them who they'd see. The esophagus is behind the heart and between the lungs. The cardiologist treats the heart and blood vessels. The pulmonologist treats the lungs and airways. Otolaryngologists (aka ENT or Ear, Nose, and Throat doctors) care for problems in the neck. In most hospitals, cardiologists, gastroenterologists, pulmonologists, and ENTs know each other and co-treat many patients. Cardiologists and pulmonologists won't treat esophagus problems, but they can tell you who to see. They won't refer you directly, but getting a name or two is invaluable.

SEE YOUR OUTPATIENT DOCTOR

Let's talk about telling your doctor.

First, make an appointment.

Then, show up!

A nurse will take you to an exam room and take your blood pressure, temperature, weight, and other measurements.

Your healthcare provider will ask why you're there. Tell them everything. They'll ask more questions, which you should answer carefully.

If you journal (among other things, it can help you remember specific esophagus attacks), bring it with you. Phillis had kept careful track of her esophagus attacks and was able to explain to her doctor in full detail about the foods that got stuck.

Don't worry if your doctor asks seemingly unrelated questions. They need to make sure it is an esophagus problem and not a heart problem or another problem. They'll ask about gastroesophageal reflux. Most patients struggling with food getting stuck also have reflux.

You mentioned chest pain, so expect questions about heart problems. For example, "Does this pain ever come on after walking or exercise?" Evaluation of cardiac disease may be necessary. For most, the pain comes after eating, not when you're walking or active. Chest pain during activity worries doctors about the heart. Chest pain after eating worries doctors about your throat or stomach. There is an overlap between cardiac-related chest pain and esophagus-related chest pain, so a cardiac evaluation (EKG and labs) may be appropriate.

Your PCP may ask you about lung problems like shortness of breath or choking. They want to make sure that the problem is related to your esophagus, and you are not choking on food. If you are choking, this is a different problem than food getting stuck in the esophagus. My approach to eating doesn't help with choking or aspirating food.

Your PCP will ask more questions. They should ask about previous abdomen or chest surgery. Your PCP will ask about cigarette smoking and alcohol. You'll learn how these habits may impact esophagus problems. Prescription drugs and your over-the-counter medications are important to know.

They will perform a physical exam, but don't be surprised if it's short. Physicians know the physical exam for swallowing problems doesn't tell us much.

After all that, your PCP will sort out different causes for your symptoms. You'll create a plan. Labs, initial medications, imaging, and referrals are part of the plan.

ALARM FEATURES

Expect these questions:

> Have you noticed weight loss since you've had this problem with eating?

> Are you experiencing dysphagia, i.e., food getting stuck while eating?

Do you have anemia?

Positive responses about unintentional weight loss, food getting stuck, and anemia are "alarm features." If you are losing weight but not trying to, physicians worry about cancer. Anemia is a lower number of red blood cells in your blood. When you have a cancer of the gastrointestinal tract, you can lose blood. A patient can easily not know they are anemic because a complete blood count is required to discover anemia.

Do these questions help doctors find patients with esophageal cancer? That's what I learned in medical school, but my experience shows me it is wrong. A large meta-analysis published in *Gastroenterology* in 2006 confirmed my experience. It looked at eighty-three different studies and 57,363 patients to see if alarm features predict cancer. In this analysis, 458 patients had cancer, so 0.8 percent of the patients had cancer. Thousands reported alarm features; it turns out, alarm features don't predict cancer.

If you've read about alarm features on Google and it paralyzed you with fear, step out of your fear cave. Your risk of cancer is 1 percent even if some of these things are true for you. Please see your doctor.

GLOBUS SENSATION

About 5 or 10 percent of my patients describe a strong sense of a lump in their throat. It can cause a feeling that food is harder to swallow or even that it gets stuck. Doctors call this the globus sensation or globus pharyngeus. The globus sensation can come after severe life stress. After my four-month-old son died from a rare heart problem, I experienced the globus sensation. It is real. You are not crazy to feel this and anyone who says that is simply wrong. It's appropriate for your PCP to ask about significant life stressors as you explain that food gets stuck.

SPEAK. YOUR. FEAR.

Before you are done with your conversation with your doctor, do something for me. Please.

Step into your fear cave and pull out the darkest, ugliest, nastiest emotion you can find. Then say it. Out loud. One sentence. Speak your fear.

Tell them how it feels. You have fears, and those fears are also part of this problem.

Here's a sampling of what I've heard. Are these familiar?

I'm scared this is cancer.

I'm afraid to eat meat.

I haven't told my husband, and I'm not sure I can.

My kids are too busy for me to bother them with this little problem.

I stopped eating out with friends five years ago because I never understand when this problem will happen, and I have to run off to the bathroom to vomit the food out.

I fear hosting holiday get-togethers. Food gets stuck when everyone is around the table. I'm not a proper host when I leave the table. I can't tell my family.

I'm worried about how much it costs to see all these doctors.

Do you know how much this test costs? How about that one?

I'm sixty-three, and I'm not on Medicare yet. I have a high-deductible health plan. All of this is coming out of my pocket.

What if speaking your fear scares you? Here are approaches that help work you up to it.

- Write it down. For your eyes only. Just writing it down gets it out and helps you process it.
- Tell your most trusted and loved person. This may be a significant other, parent, adult child, religious figure, etc.
- Combo special: write down your fear and share the written version with your most trusted and loved person.

- Share on social media. For some, sharing on social media feels anonymous and easier than sharing with family. For others, sharing with family is easier.

No matter where you share your fear, help yourself work toward speaking your fear to another human. Then work up to sharing it with your healthcare provider.

I'll never forget the patient who came to see me because food was getting stuck. Angelina was ninety-five years old and had periodic esophagus attacks. She had poor vision, was hard of hearing, and used a wheelchair, though she could stand for a minute or two.

Angelina tells me she hasn't eaten solid food for months and wants to know if she'll ever eat "people food" again. My heart sank, hearing my patient tell me she didn't even feel like a person anymore.

Frail as she seemed, Angelina made it through an esophagram okay. It showed she had a long narrowing or stricture of her esophagus, which I explain to her. She needed to see a GI doctor to dilate her esophagus, which would take at least five days to set up. I was almost afraid to ask her the question I always save for last: *how does all this make you feel?* But I do, and the tears stream from her eyes and her voice cracks as she answers. I don't even really need the words to understand her.

POP QUIZ

Q. Which healthcare providers can you tell about food getting stuck?

1. Gastroenterologist

2. Any MD/DO physician

3. Any mid-level provider (NP, PA, APRN, etc.)

4. Speech therapist

5. Any of the above

Answer: 5. Any of the above.

Helping Angelina heal was going to take more than a balloon and some pills. More on those options to come, but I'm a strong believer that every successful doctor-patient relationship will need to take into account how the health problems affect the emotions, not just the physical body.

If speaking your fear resonates, read Philip McKernan's book, *One Last Talk*. He lays out a simple method to share your most important truth with those you love. He says, "Your greatest gift lies next to your deepest wound." So true. But don't let reading another book keep you from seeking medical help.

LABS

Phyllis' doctor ordered a panel of different lab tests. She got an IV. In other words, a needle pokes into a vein in her arm to remove blood. Lab tests often require that you have not eaten for eight hours or overnight. So, you will need another lab appointment time. Usually, this is in the morning. A complete blood count (CBC) and a comprehensive metabolic panel are both appropriate. Other lab tests may be necessary, depending on your specific complaint and history. If you are seeing a gastroenterologist, there may be additional lab tests they order.

INITIAL MEDICATIONS

Your healthcare provider will probably tell you to take an over-the-counter medication or give you a medication prescription for a pharmacy. Phyllis' doctor prescribed a proton pump inhibitor (PPI), which is the most common choice. You will learn more about PPIs in chapter 11. Please take them as prescribed. My most important message about PPIs is they do not stop reflux. PPIs make the gastric secretions less acidic. Less stomach acid means less esophagus damage. The PPIs do not make the sphincter squeeze better. Many patients tell me they stop the PPI because they felt the reflux sensation while taking the medicine. You need to change eating behavior to prevent reflux. Chapter 9 discusses this further. Your doctor wants to know if your pain improves after thirty days. Some call this the thirty-day omeprazole test. Take-home message: please take the medications your doctor recommends.

INITIAL IMAGING

Some doctors recommend a radiology swallowing test before you see a GI doctor. Imaging is less expensive and less invasive than endoscopy. The exams are called an esophagram or an upper GI (gastrointestinal) exam. A radiologist takes pictures of your proximal GI tract to look for problems. These pictures form a roadmap of your esophagus and stomach and help the GI doctor better understand your problem. This is where I met Phyllis. Your PCP may order this, or your gastroenterologist may ask for it. My advice: roll with it either way.

BARIUM STUDY (ESOPHAGRAM OR UPPER GI)

I've performed between 1,000-10,000 radiology exams of the esophagus. I'll tell you enough to reduce fear and anxiety but not overload you.

Don't eat for four to eight hours. You stand in an X-ray room. You drink an effervescent agent with water followed by contrast. An effervescent agent is something that creates gas. It's the most carbonated beverage you've ever drunk. It reminds me of Alka-Seltzer, if you've ever had one of those. The contrast tastes thick and chalky. Sometimes it's flavored—

vanilla, banana, cherry, and strawberry might be options. It's unpleasant but not awful.

The radiologist or their assistant takes pictures of your esophagus, stomach, and other parts of your bowel. It takes five to fifteen minutes. You'll swallow a 12.7 mm (1/2 inch) pill.

Swallowing this pill is the bar test (as in barium tablet test). The bar test checks for a narrowing of your esophagus called a stricture. If the pill passes, fantastic! That means your esophagus is at least 12.7 mm in diameter, and food bites of this size or smaller will pass. If the pill gets stuck, it signals a problem. Many patients tell me when the tablet gets stuck, it replicates their symptoms. Unfortunately, endoscopy misses esophagus strictures. One study estimated 75 percent of the narrowings were overlooked. Because of this, the Bar Test helps us detect more strictures and guide the GI doctors to them. We discover many things on this exam, but the Bar Test is an essential step for patients if food gets stuck. After the exam, the radiologist creates a report for your doctor. As medical tests go, this is easy. Phyllis wasn't a fan of the contrast, but she was in and out in thirty minutes. She didn't need a driver and enjoyed a late breakfast with a friend afterward.

Another imaging exam is ultrasound. Right upper quadrant ultrasound or an ultrasound abdomen helps discover other causes of pain. Sound waves help us see parts of your upper abdomen. You don't eat for four to eight hours. An ultra-sound technologist takes pictures of the organs in your belly. Your gallbladder can be a source of pain after eating. As medical exams go, ultrasounds are easy.

LESS VALUABLE IMAGING EXAMS

What *not* to do is sometimes as important as what *to* do. If you have pain after eating, a head CT or brain MRI is not part of the initial evaluation. An MRI of any part of the body would not be reasonable. If the first round of testing (esopha-gram, ultrasound, and endoscopy) are normal, a CT scan of the abdomen and pelvis with contrast is next. If you are one of the 1 percent who has esophageal cancer, a CT of the chest, abdomen, and pelvis with contrast becomes a necessary exam. Another less valuable exam is a small bowel follow-through. For this exam, you drink contrast, and we take pictures of your gut after the stomach to the colon. Small bowel exams don't help people with problems swallowing.

There's one more swallowing exam. It goes by different names: modified barium swallow, video swallowing study, or videofluoroscopic swallowing exam. This test looks for liquid or solid food entering your trachea, called aspiration. The trachea is also known as the windpipe and leads to your lungs. Liquid or food going into your windpipe or lungs is a lousy thing that can be treated. If you think you "choke" on your food, this exam looks for that. You sit in a chair while you eat different foods mixed with barium. A speech pathologist watches you swallow while a radiologist administers X-rays. We take pictures of your mouth and throat from the side to make sure everything you swallow goes to the right place.

Most patients who describe food getting stuck don't have this test. But, if you do choke on food, this is the test for you.

REFERRALS
GI

Your PCP will ask other doctors for help and their advice. A gastroenterologist is typically first on the list. They are the physicians who take care of the esophagus, stomach, and the rest of the GI tract. During my career, GI doctors have been a joy and luxury to work together with to help patients. When you see a GI doctor, they'll ask you a host of questions about your problem. They will order lab tests and other GI tests we'll discuss later in this chapter. However, some smaller towns don't have enough people to support a gastroenterologist. In smaller towns, you may see a general surgeon or a family physician. As a patient, you may need to choose between receiving your care more conveniently locally or traveling to see a specialist.

For more than 80 percent of Americans, you live within thirty miles of a GI doctor. That's who I see for help.

ENT

An otolaryngologist (aka, ENT or Ear, Nose, and Throat doctor) may be asked for help. If you feel like food sticks in your neck rather than your chest, the likelihood you see an ENT doctor rises. Just like a GI doctor, they'll ask many questions about your problem. They are experts in the neck. Like GI doctors, ENTs may not practice in a smaller community.

CARDIOLOGY

You might be referred to a cardiologist. This doctor cares for patients with heart problems. If you see a cardiologist, they will ask similar questions to what is previously in this chapter. They will probably do an EKG, which is a study of the electrical impulse system of your heart. The cardiologist will also likely perform some sort of stress-based exam to see how well your heart reacts to exercise. A stress EKG, stress echocardiogram, or another stress-based imaging study tests for heart problems during exercise.

PULMONARY

Your PCP may send you to a pulmonologist. Pulmonologists help patients with breathing problems. They focus on your lungs and airways. What do the lungs have to do with swallowing? Some patients with GER (gastroesophageal reflux) also have chronic pneumonia (infection of the lungs). The patient sleeps, refluxes stomach acid upward, aspirates it into their lungs, and causes pneumonia. Asthma in adults and children may be related to reflux. The pulmonologist helps treat lung problems related to reflux.

NEUROLOGY

It would be unusual for you to see a neurologist about esophagus problems. These physicians specialize in the nervous system. Think of the nervous system as the electrical communication system between our brain, spinal cord, hands, feet, and the organs of our body. Chapter 12 explores this further, but nerve-based diseases can cause esophagus problems called motility disorders. Nerve-based problems represent less than 10 percent of swallowing problems. The most common nerve-based problem with swallowing comes from a stroke of the brain. If you have had a stroke, you probably know a neurologist. They treat patients with strokes, reduce their risk of future strokes, and treat other nerve-based diseases.

GI TESTS

The initial exam for the GI doctor is upper endoscopy. I discussed it in chapter 3 in the Endoscopy Lab section.

The ENT doctor offers a similar exam called transnasal esophagoscopy (TNE). You sit upright in an exam chair. Your ENT doctor sprays a strong anesthetic into your nose and throat to numb the surface. Then they pass a spaghetti-sized tube with a light and camera on the end through your nose. Since they don't pass through the mouth, you shouldn't gag. Because only numbing medicine is used, you're awake and can watch if you want. It takes less time (about twenty minutes) than upper endoscopy and because there's no sedation, you can return to work afterward. Small pieces of abnormal tissue (biopsies) can be removed during TNE.

The GI doctor performs other exams that I'll explain.

PH PROBE TESTING

pH probe testing (i.e., ambulatory pH monitoring, twenty-four to forty-eight-hour pH monitoring) is an exam performed by the GI doctor. pH is a measure of how acidic or how basic a substance is. pH takes many back to high school chemistry, but let's keep it simple. The pH scale ranges from 1 to 14. Distilled water is neutral at 7.0. The acid secreted by your stomach has a pH of around 2.0. A pH probe or capsule is a medical device placed into your distal esophagus to measure pH.

If the pH probe detects a pH below 4.0 (i.e., 3.9 down to 1.0), the GI doctor assumes gastric acid refluxed into your esophagus. You must avoid acidic beverages, for example, Coke (2.5), Sprite (3.3), grapefruit juice (3.8), and apple juice (3.4) while pH probe testing. Drink water during pH probe testing. Monitoring lasts twenty-four or forty-eight hours while you eat your normal diet. Many pH systems allow you to click a button if you feel reflux or pain. Recording these episodes helps the GI doctor see if your pH drops or you have reflux at the same time as you have pain. Some consider pH probe testing the best test for GERD.

MANOMETRY

Manometry (i.e., high-resolution manometry or HRM) tests how well the esophagus muscles contract. They start by numbing up your nose and throat. Then a catheter is advanced through your nose down your esophagus. Advancing the catheter may be mildly uncomfortable for a few seconds, then you're usually okay. While testing, you drink sips of water every twenty or thirty seconds. Then thirty-six sensors measure the pressure in your esophagus. GI doctors pay careful attention to the proximal and distal esophagus pressures. The pressure waves created as the esophagus muscles contract and relax is also important. Manometry is performed upright, partially upright, or sometimes lying down. If your esophagus muscles don't contract well, manometry helps GI doctors uncover this problem. Doctors call these problems with muscle contraction motility disorders. Manometry helps sort out the different motility disorders. There are many books dedicated to the different motility problems. I won't dig into all the problems here.

COSTS

Books are written about healthcare costs in the USA and around the world. This book won't touch those complicated issues. Here's a table of what different hospitals charge for procedures. I included an estimate of what Medicare pays doctors and/or hospitals for the same procedures. These are gross estimates of hospital charges and Medicare reimbursement for these exams. Actual reimbursement depends on where you live, malpractice insurance costs, and many other factors.

The amount hospitals and doctors charge patients varies massively around the country.

If you want to find out exactly how much a hospital charges for a procedure, you can find it. On January 1, 2019, Medicare required hospitals to post their charges online. If you Google your hospital's name and "Master Charge List" you'll find a large spreadsheet to download. Warning: it's opaque and challenging. The 800-bed tertiary care medical center included 65,585 items. The 600-bed quaternary care center listed 45,636 items. A 200-bed regional hospital listed 7,807 items. The same exam at these four sites may be called four different things. A hospital-based upper endoscopy is called an EGD and the large hospitals list over ten different variants on the EGD. Compiling this table took me over four hours and assistance from medical billing experts.

You might have better luck finding missing needles in haystacks than uncovering healthcare costs from master charge lists. Good luck!

EXAM	CPT CODE (IF APPLICABLE)	QUATERNARY MEDICAL CENTER 1/1/2019 (EST OR ACTUAL)	TERTIARY MEDICAL CENTER 1/1/20 (ESTIMATE OR ACTUAL)	REGIONAL MEDICAL CENTER 1/1/20	OUTPATIENT CLINIC CHARGES 1/1/20	MEDICARE REIMBURSES IN 2020 (ACTUAL OR CLOSE ESTIMATE)
PCP H&P HB PREVENTIVE VISIT, NEW, 18 - 39	99385	N/A	$389	N/A	$192	$209
SPECIALIST CONSULT (SEEING A GI DOCTOR)	99204	N/A	$389	N/A	$218	$209
ESOPHAGRAM	74220	$1,967	$648	$421	$312	$103
ULTRASOUND RIGHT UPPER QUADRANT	76700	$2,059	$780	$740	$411	$57
CT ABDOMEN AND PELVIS	74177	$10,437	$5,082	$5,137	$1,000	$198
OTC PPI 30D SUPPLY	N/A	N/A	N/A	N/A	N/A	$60
OTC H2-BLOCKER 30D SUPPLY	N/A	N/A	N/A	N/A	N/A	$20
RX PPI 30 DAY SUPPLY	N/A	N/A	N/A	N/A	N/A	$200
PH PROBE MONITORING		Unknown	$2,205	Not offered.	Not offered.	$455
HIGH-RESOLUTION MANOMETRY		$2,554	$1,754	Not offered.	Not offered.	$455

EXAM	CPT CODE (IF APPLICABLE)	QUATERNARY MEDICAL CENTER 1/1/2019 (EST OR ACTUAL)	TERTIARY MEDICAL CENTER 1/1/20 (ESTIMATE OR ACTUAL)	REGIONAL MEDICAL CENTER 1/1/20	OUTPATIENT CLINIC CHARGES 1/1/20	MEDICARE REIMBURSES IN 2020 (ACTUAL OR CLOSE ESTIMATE)
FLIP		$3,142	$2,219	Not offered.	Not Offered.	$455
ECG/EKG	93000	$1,214	$56	$264	$45	$50
2 VIEW CHEST X-RAY	71020	$872	$390	$347	$100	$20
IV GLUCAGON		$1,139	$772	"Variable"	N/A	$145
ER PHYSICIAN CHARGE LEVEL 5		$11,522	$2,966	$1,804	N/A	$209
ENDOSCOPY HOSPITAL-BASED		$7,281	$1,960	$2,247	N/A	$1,813
ENDOSCOPY DILATION		$7,281	$3,289		N/A	$1,813

Congratulations! You completed your esophagus fellowship, and now have a good grasp on what to expect from physicians' visits for problems swallowing! Before you go on to learn some of the self-help strategies you can employ, I'll leave you with some answers for Phyllis.

Phyllis's labs were normal. Her esophagram showed mild reflux, a small hiatal hernia, and a benign stricture. Her GI doctor recommended a PPI for thirty days and took a look inside her esophagus with a camera and dilated it. Now, Phyllis swallows normally again. Her pain is gone. Anxiety, uncertainty, and fear disappeared. Her esophagus problem is gone, and the inner emotional turmoil that came with it is gone, too. Phyllis knows to see the doctor without delay if this ever happens again, and feels confident she'll be helped.

As we've discussed, working with a healthcare provider is absolutely critical. That doesn't mean there aren't important strategies to learn to rescue yourself from stuck food and avoid an esophagus attack in the first place. That's what's coming up next in part 2.

PART 2

THREE STEPS TO ENJOY EATING AGAIN

CHAPTER 5

KNOW WHAT TO DO WHEN FOOD IS STUCK

During residency, my wife and I loved to go out for dinner. One of our favorites was a Thai place, and we loved their signature dish, Crispy Red Curry Duck.

One of our nights there, I was *famished*. So when the duck arrived, I dug right in to quell my hunger.

In my hurry, of course, it sticks. Right in the middle of date night!

Abraham Lincoln long ago said, "He who represents himself has a fool for a client." The same rings true for physicians. When we attempt to self-diagnosis or treat family members, layers of bias prevent an accurate diagnosis.

I had official training in the anatomy and process underlying this problem, and my understanding had grown over the years; yet still, I struggled to put it together and apply it to *myself*. I forgot my eating rules when hungry.

That night, it took only sips of water, patience, relaxation, and walking outside the restaurant to get the duck to pass. Eventually, I swallowed gulps of water to prove to myself the duck passed into my stomach, and I went back to the rest of my meal…carefully. It isn't always accomplished as easily, I know from hard experience. But it can be done!

What do you do when you swallow something, it sticks, and you're in pain? What to do, RIGHT NOW! Pain, frustration, and anxiety collide, and you experience a crescendo of fear. I know—I've been there. Don't let fear take over. I can't begin to count my esophagus attacks over the last eighteen years.

I'll explain the process I take the second I feel an esophagus attack come on.

I'll sprinkle in stories to help reinforce the principles. We'll discuss guardrails about when to contact 911 or visit your local emergency room.

How do you know food is stuck?

I have my own stories, but I'm just one person. Patients have told me hundreds of stories over the last eighteen years. The stories vary, but common themes emerge.

Patients feel food stuck and most point to a fleshy spot right above their sternum where their neck meets their chest. This is the top of the lightning bolt on the front cover. Seventy to eighty percent of my patients tell me about chest pain. Some point to where their lower sternum meets their abdomen and describe pain there. That's the lower point of the front cover lightning bolt. They describe a squeezing pain that comes on in waves that last three to five seconds. Most patients express no desire to eat more solid food when something is stuck. (Which is good, because you shouldn't.)

YOU'RE NOT CHOKING

I need to make an important distinction.

Food stuck in your esophagus is not choking. Two openings are in your throat. A flap of tissue that acts like a valve called the epiglottis. Muscles close the epiglottis when you swallow and cover the trachea. Your trachea is the tube air passes through to your lungs. As you eat, the epiglottis closes, covers the trachea, and food passes into the esophagus. If the epiglottis doesn't close or you try to talk and swallow, food can get stuck at the epiglottis and cause choking. Choking is food getting stuck in the airway, not the esophagus. These are two distinct problems.

Choking on food is an emergency. It makes it harder or impossible to breathe. You may hear audible wheezing. You should put your hands around your neck to signal you are choking and signal that you need someone to do the Heimlich maneuver. If you're alone, try performing the Heimlich maneuver with a table or chair. You will pass out in one to two minutes if food blocks your trachea, and human brain cells start to die four to six minutes later.

Other things get stuck in the esophagus. Over 99 percent of the time, it's food that obstructs. Or a bone can get stuck. Fish and chicken bones are the most common. *If a bone obstructs, proceed to an emergency department. Do not try to pass a bone on your own.*

If you take only one piece of information from this chapter, here it is: **stop eating solid food if something is stuck.**

I divide solid food into two categories in chapter 7: easy solids and difficult solids. Easy solids you *know* will pass. For most people, this is corn kernels, green peas, most beans, non-sticky rice, pudding, and yogurt. Easy solids are small or near-liquid. Difficult solids are foods that could block your esophagus. If food is stuck, don't eat solid food. No easy solids. No difficult solids.

Why? No patient has ever told me eating more solid food helped. It never works for me. In fact, every time I try to eat more solid food while something is stuck, it causes more problems.

Doctors give patients medicines that relax the esophagus along with liquid and gas to help food pass. My analogy is stacking stones in a plastic tube. The first stone is your first piece of food stuck in your esophagus. Food stuck causes esophagus muscles to contract and relax to help the food pass. Your esophagus doesn't like food stuck. A second piece of food stacks upon the first and exerts twice the weight upon the first piece of food at the point of obstruction. Stacking more things in the esophagus makes it contract stronger. The intense contractions cause you more pain—pain I call the esophagus attack. None of this helps food pass. Liquid is the answer.

LIQUID FIRST

When food feels stuck, take a small sip of liquid first. I prefer carbonated water over tap or still water, but any form of water is best. In the ER, we only give patients 30 mL of water. That's about one ounce of water or two tablespoons. A shot glass of water. A small sip. Not a gulp. Never chug. More is not better here.

When you take a small sip and food is stuck, it causes pain. Your esophagus muscle contracts, relaxes, and even spasms against the obstruction. If there's any opening, liquid will pass. Think about a beaver dam. Water always finds any hole in the dam and gets through. The liquid adds lubrication at the blockage (more on this in chapter 6). As liquid passes and your esophagus contracts and relaxes, the food blockage may wiggle forward. Sometimes, water works right away. Other times, it takes a few small sips. I space out sips every thirty to sixty seconds. Follow your pain experience to try more liquid or wait. If it still hurts, wait. If the pain goes away, try another small sip.

What is the difference between a 95 percent obstruction and a 100 percent obstruction? If food totally obstructs and I take a small sip, pain increases and doesn't let off after sixty seconds. If I take another small sip, the pain is worse, and I feel a new fullness in my chest. It is hard to explain besides unrelenting pain and increasing fullness. If I'm 95 percent obstructed, the pain comes on for fifteen to thirty seconds and lets up. When I take my next small sip, I have pain like the first pain episode that lasts fifteen to thirty seconds but dissipates. If you're continuing to take more sips and the pain is worsening, stop taking sips. Go to your emergency room.

CARBONATED WATER WORKS BETTER THAN TAP WATER

Remember the effervescent agent makes gas in chapter 3? Water and gas are two ingredients used in emergency rooms to pass obstructed food. Remember, 56 percent of patients passed the food blockage with an effervescent agent and water? Carbonated beverages are one of your best tools to help advance stuck food. I rarely drink tap water at meals. If a meal includes difficult solids, I have liquid handy—more on this in chapters 6 and 8.

I met Pam at a small hospital in rural Iowa. Pam described esophagus attacks, and she was a lifelong Coke drinker. When her doctor told her losing weight helps reflux, Pam set out in a new direction. Pam switched from Coke to carbonated water, which had the advantage of being lower acid as well as lower calorie. Tap water bores her, so Pam only drinks flavored carbonated water—key lime is her favorite—at meals because it helps her pass obstructed food. I congratulated Pam because she successfully lost five pounds switching from a sugary, acidic Coke to zero-calorie flavored water. I love Pam's healthy substitution and her weight loss. I doubly love that the carbonated beverage helps Pam pass food while eating. Win-win scenarios are the best.

Patients ask about beer or other carbonated alcohols like champagne. They work, but they're not my first choice. Beer works if you don't have carbonated water. It's carbonated liquid, so it helps. I prefer water. Don't use wine or hard alcohol to help food pass. More potent alcohol with prolonged contact with your esophagus may damage it.

STAND UP

After drinking carbonated water, I move to my next step. I stand up.

If I stand up during a meal, my wife always asks, "Something stuck?" She knows as well as I do what getting out of my chair mid-meal means.

My second most important lesson of this chapter is: **you need to tell your significant other.** Come up with a plan now. My verbal answer of "Yes" assures her I'm not choking. You must tell your significant other so they don't confuse this with choking.

Standing up does one thing: it straightens the esophagus. Many people slump while eating. Standing up straightens everything out.

There is only a small one- to five-degree change in orientation. Maybe it helps 3 percent of the time?

My patient Rose told me a story that highlights the need to tell your significant other about the problem.

Rose experienced an esophagus attack. She stood up from the table and grimaced in pain, fist clenched in front of her chest. Rose's loving husband didn't know what was going on but suspected the worst. He rushed to her, wrapped his arms around his wife, and performed the Heimlich maneuver. He thought he was saving her life.

Only Rose wasn't choking. So the Heimlich didn't help. Worse, it actually put her at risk. Rose's husband's Heimlich was textbook. Meaning, he compressed her lower ribcage hard with an upward thrust. The Heimlich maneuver squeezes air out of the lungs and violently expels food from the windpipe. Rose's husband might have (but fortunately didn't) broken her ribs and caused more problems.

You don't want to find yourself in Rose's position! Tell your significant other food gets stuck, so they understand. Make sure there's no confusion between choking and an esophagus attack.

BURP

After standing, my next maneuver is burping.

One reason for standing is so you can walk out of the room and burp. When you burp, you release air from your stomach and esophagus from your mouth. You can burp quietly or loudly. Burping air opens the distal esophagus. Burping air may reorient or even move the obstructed food. Blocked food can be any shape. Burping may move it enough that your esophagus can pass it. Burping helps me maybe 10 percent of the time.

When Thai duck was stuck in my esophagus, I got up from the table, walked away, and burped several times. The pain improved—the burping was probably shifting the position of the duck in my esophagus to help it pass.

SIP LIQUID AGAIN

Once I've burped once or twice, I drink a sip of carbonated water again. Don't worry that burping is releasing gas from the carbonated beverage. It is. That's okay. Burping and drinking small sips of liquid work together. Beware a return of pain after each little swallow. It should last fifteen to thirty seconds and stop. **Pain lasting longer than a minute signals a complete food blockage and is a red flag to go to an emergency room.**

Does this scare you? I get that. I'm presenting strategies developed over eighteen years and thousands of esophagus attacks. In other words, you can't just snap your fingers and solve this problem. If food is stuck and this worries you, causes fear, you don't know how to burp, or you don't understand, that's okay. If you're overwhelmed, you need a doctor's help.

My goal is for you to be more comfortable, more knowledgeable, and more empowered. If you're overwhelmed, you need a doctor's help. Go to a hospital.

RELAXATION BREATHING

After burping, my next maneuver is to calm myself with relaxation breathing.

This is hard. I get it.

I've been there. FOOD IS STUCK! I CANNOT CALM DOWN! IT HURTS!

If you know you cannot calm yourself down, then skip this part. If you can, I want you to spend thirty to sixty seconds with relaxed breathing. Yoga breathing is best. Relaxing your mind by thinking about something calming helps, too. Try a three-second slow breath in through your nose and a four-second breath out of your mouth. Repeat that cycle five to ten times.

As I breathe, my mind goes to the treed woods behind our home. It's a dense hilly wooded area where I take relaxing walks.

Your calm relaxing place might be a beach somewhere. It might be your favorite massage table. For some, it's an easy run or cross-country skiing. Wherever you go for relaxation, mentally go there now and breathe.

I don't want deep breaths because big pressure changes in your chest might squeeze your esophagus too much.

Take slow, relaxed, easy breaths. Relaxation is your goal. When you're relaxed, your esophagus muscles relax. Remember how glucagon relaxes the esophagus? We give it to patients in the emergency room to relax the esophagus. Same idea. With easy breathing and relaxing visualization, you're trying to relax the esophagus muscle to help food pass. Calm breathing, walking outside the restaurant, and relaxing myself helped me pass the duck from my esophagus.

Relaxation and breathing exercises are hard if you're in pain or anxious. Now for a straightforward request. Don't go back to the table. I don't want you tempted to eat more solid food. When this happens to me, I get a small glass of water and bring it with me.

Don't return to the table.

Don't tempt yourself to eat more solid food until the obstruction passes.

I often ask patients if they can tell when the obstructed food has passed. Patients tell me the same story.

Patient: "Dr. Lake, it's so easy to tell. The [_____] goes away. Instantly."

For some patients, that blank says "pain."

Others say, "fullness," "the sensation," or "the squeezing feeling."

Every patient tells me something like, "You just know." They describe the relief. When relief happens, or the pain passes, let your entire body relax.

Stop the eating process and enjoy the relief that comes from overcoming this problem for a minute.

Remind yourself that you can overcome this problem with understanding and knowledge.

What if no relief comes? Or the pain improves, but you're not sure anything passed. Can you tell the blockage passed if you don't feel it?

Take a test sip of water.

If it goes down fine, take a little larger sip. Then a gulp.

If that's working, try consecutive swallows. Once you've proven the food blockage has passed, you may return to solid food.

VALSALVA MANEUVER

My next strategy is the Valsalva maneuver. You've done a

Valsalva maneuver thousands of times and didn't know it. The Valsalva maneuver doesn't work for me, but a few patients tell me it works. Take in a slight breath, close your mouth and throat, and try to breathe out. You've now done a Valsalva maneuver. Here's a more specific example of a Valsalva maneuver. When you go to the bathroom and bear down to defecate (i.e., pass stool), you are also performing a Valsalva maneuver. Don't strain as much as you do with a bowel movement. A forceful Valsalva maneuver raises the pressure in your chest about 40 mmHg. This increased pressure pushes on your esophagus.

Resting pressure in the lower esophagus sphincter is 20 mmHg, so raising it to 40 mmHg may help pass food.

When your esophagus is contracting and relaxing, and trying to pass obstructed food, the pressure is higher.

Often, the pressure is much higher. In chapter 3, you learned about manometry. Manometry measures pressure in the esophagus. Your esophagus generates pressures over 100 mmHg when it contracts. When food sticks for me, the Valsalva maneuver doesn't help. My theory is the 40 mmHg generated during Valsalva doesn't overcome the 100 mmHg pressure of a contracting esophagus. But some patients tell me the Valsalva maneuver helps.

In seventy-five volunteers, one article found that the pressure at the junction of the stomach and esophagus was 5 mmHg but varied by 17 mmHg depending on breathing. This confirms what patients tell me that manipulating their breathing and performing a Valsalva maneuver may help pass obstructed food from their esophagus.

Ninety-nine percent of you will have no problem doing a Valsalva maneuver. If you bear down for bowel movements with no problem, you have no worries. A powerful Valsalva treats some abnormal heart rhythms. If you have severe congestive heart failure (i.e., CHF), you should check with your doctor before attempting a powerful Valsalva.

VOMITING

What if nothing works? What if sips of liquid, standing up, burping, relaxing my body, relaxing my breathing, and a Valsalva maneuver fail? You have two choices. One, go to an emergency room. Two, retch and vomit the obstructed food. Patients are embarrassed to admit to me that they do this.

I always assure them it's okay, and medically it is safe. (I hate doing it, myself, but what works, works.)

911 OR EMERGENCY ROOM

Go to the ER if vomiting fails.

Please do not worry if this happens.

It happens every day—over 65,000 per year in the USA. That is just about 178 people each day!

WHEW! IT PASSED! NOW WHAT?

What if food passes? What if one of these strategies works? You have homework. First, appreciate your success. Obstructed food passed.

Give yourself a silent high five. Seriously, this is an important part of the process. Relax and be grateful. You're learning strategies that help with this problem and acknowledge your success. Don't forget that you saved an emergency room bill!

Step 1: After the obstruction passes, acknowledge your success.

Step 2: Return to the table and tell your partner the food passed. Do not overlook *their* worry and anxiety. They want to make sure you're okay.

Step 3: Look at your plate. Try to figure out what caused the obstruction. How big was the piece of food?

Recall your last bite and what got stuck. Don't retake the same bite. You will eat the same food on your plate again, but you will take a different approach. Chapters 6-8 spell out my

3-step strategy to avoid food getting stuck. That's next. I fill chapter II with strategies to help you conquer difficult solids.

Let's review the essential chapter takeaways:

When food gets stuck, don't eat more solid food!

Liquid only.

Tell someone nearby.

Stand up.

Burp.

Try liquid again.

POP QUIZ

Q. *What's the worst thing you can do when food is stuck?*

1. Take small sips of liquid.

2. Tell someone about your problem.

3. Stand up.

4. Eat more of what got stuck and hope it fixes itself.

Answer: 4. NEVER eat more solid food when something is stuck.

Try to relax.

Consider a Valsalva maneuver or vomiting.

Go to an emergency room if nothing helps.

This list worked for me during The Night of the Crispy Red Curry Duck. When I went back to my dinner and my wife, I doubled-down on my efforts to cut up my food more, chew more, and take my time. That's the kind of strategy we'll dive into in the next chapter: learning to avoid food getting stuck in the first place.

AFTER FOOD PASSES HOMEWORK

HIGH-FIVE	Acknowledge your success.
TELL YOUR PARTNER	Let the other person in your life know, so they aren't anxious.
ASSESS LAST SOLID BITE	Figure out what got stuck, why it got stuck, and don't eat the same bite again.

CHAPTER 6

LIQUID BEFORE
SOLID

Olivia was serving her cat some deli sliced turkey for breakfast—lucky cat!—and decided to share the meal. But as soon
as she swallowed, she felt a painful squeezing sensation in
her chest. She was caught so off-guard she knocked the cat's
dish right off the counter.

She grabbed the closest thing she thought would wash it
down: milk. A little sip, and, hallelujah, the pain released. It
felt like the turkey had passed along its journey, as originally
planned. Relief! Another sip of milk went down fine on its
own, then a gulp. Olivia felt her body, which had been on
high-alert a moment ago, relax. She felt completely better,
though she was a little wary of eating again. The whole episode was too alarming, and Olivia immediately made an
appointment to see her doctor.

Olivia's doctor heard her story and sent her on to me for an esophagram. Olivia relayed the whole tale to me, still trying to make sense of it for herself. How had a slice of turkey— *thin-sliced* turkey—gotten stuck when chunks of steak went down fine at dinner the night before?

While I explained my 3-step process, Olivia released frustration and fear. As Olivia learned how the esophagus works, what happens when it doesn't, and how to help it keep working 100 percent, she visibly relaxed in her face and body. She released concerns and confusion and gained confidence over the problem with a natural system.

Where she'd already begun to worry about not knowing when food would get stuck, and fear of eating at family gatherings, or out with friends, or at favorite restaurants, she traded those worries for the sense of control that comes with knowledge and understanding.

Olivia had instinctively tried my Step 1—Liquid Before Solid—without even knowing any doctor might recommend it. And if she remembered nothing else from our conversation that would have been a good lesson to take with her: her instinct to take small sips of liquid were spot-on.

There are two reasons Liquid Before Solid works.

1. Liquid and saliva coat your esophagus and make it slicker. Food passes easier.
2. Swallowing tells your spinal cord and brain you're eating. Nerves send signals to your esophagus muscles, "Open and close! Contract and relax!"

Humans average 600 swallows per day, and many are saliva. We make 1-1.5 L of saliva a day. Saliva is 98 percent water, but other things in saliva moisturize and lubricate your mouth and throat. Your salivary glands make saliva and help with swallowing. Besides lubricating the esophagus, liquid seldom gets stuck in the esophagus. I do have one warning, which I'll get to a bit later, but you can generally consider liquid safe.

Swallowing liquid also "wakes up the esophagus," as I explain it to patients. When you sit down for a meal, your brain knows you're about to eat. But your esophagus is a muscle. It doesn't know you're about to eat until it gets a message from your brain.

Sipping alerts your esophagus that liquid, and later food, is coming. A complex neural network jumps into action when you swallow. Swallowing liquid signals your spinal cord. Your spinal cord relays signals further down your esophagus. These signals tell your esophagus to open. Gulping or consecutive swallows cascades more alerts to your esophagus muscles to prepare for more. The muscles contract, relax, and move liquid along to the stomach.

WARMING UP

What's your sport or physical activity? Golfing, skiing, running, walking, swimming, weightlifting? Whatever your favorite, I bet it comes with a warm-up strategy. Few golfers walk on the course, skip the practice range, skip the warm-up, and skip the practice swings. I'm not a golfer, but I've never heard of someone walking onto the course and ripping off a 300-yard drive without a warm-up. No runner walks out the door for a max effort 5K or timed mile without jogging or active stretching.

Your esophagus is a muscle like other muscles in your body. My 3-step strategy relies on warming up the esophagus before we challenge it. Eating steak or other difficult solids is challenging for our esophagus. Our first step to warm-up is…(say it with me) Liquid Before Solid.

WHAT LIQUID IS BEST?

Patients often ask what liquid is best.

Carbonated mineral water with a pH above 5.0 (not too acidic) is my favorite.

Tap water or iced tea are great choices.

Carbonated alcoholic beverages? Beer works.

POP QUIZ

Q. Which of these choices is best to warm up your esophagus before a meal?

1. Hot tea.

2. Whiskey.

3. Tap water.

4. Egg nog.

Answer: 3. Tap water. Of these choices, tap water is my choice.

I caution about hot beverages. Ever gotten coffee from a drive-through? The coffee is too hot. Even a tiny sip burns my tongue. Scalding your esophagus is NOT the warm-up strategy we're looking for here! We need to take small sips. Moderate-sized swallows, then gulps to warm up your esophagus.

Patients ask about thicker consistency liquids and whether they help with the warm-up process. Orange juice and milk are thicker or more viscous than water. They work great; just ask Olivia after her episode with thin-sliced turkey. Thin kefir? Great, too.

A smoothie or thick shake isn't as good. A thick shake or a protein smoothie isn't liquid. It's closer to ice cream, and it can get stuck. It doesn't help the warm-up process.

WHAT IF I CAN'T DRINK LIQUIDS?

Here's my warning about thin liquids. Some patients aspirate thin liquids into their lungs. Aspiration is when liquid doesn't go into your esophagus, and the liquid ends up in your trachea (aka, windpipe) and your lungs. The most common cause is a stroke. Dementia, Parkinson's disease, and multiple sclerosis (MS) are also causes. If a speech therapist or physician says avoid thin liquids, honor their recommendation. Your speech therapist or physician will help you discover safe liquids. The form of liquid they recommend you drink (nectar consistency, honey consistency, etc.) is what you must use.

Xerostomia means dry mouth. If you make less saliva, you need to drink more liquid to compensate. Drinking plenty of liquid helps you eat, especially if you have dry mouth. Knowledge is power, and you can overcome this.

Remember chapter 1 when the turkey got stuck, and I thought I had a heart attack? I had broken rule #1 (before I even knew it was rule #1): I downed the turkey before any liquid. I needed liquid first to coat, lubricate, and warm up my esophagus. Now, when Olivia feeds her cat, she knows to drink milk, orange juice, or water before she shares turkey slices. Olivia and I taught you rule #1: liquid before solid!

This is a first easy step to avoiding getting "stuck." And we also know sipping liquid can work to get something that feels stuck to pass. I hope you will allow your growing knowledge to relieve not only your physical symptoms but also the emotions associated with them. Name your fears. Tell someone you love about releasing them and plan how you'll celebrate success.

But before you get too carried away, don't forget to make the other two steps your own, starting with the next chapter, for Step 2.

CHAPTER 7

EASY SOLIDS BEFORE DIFFICULT SOLIDS

Having all my kids and grandkids together for lunch on Easter is a joy to my soul. It's more than worth all the cooking beforehand, and all the dishes that will follow. We clink our glasses and toast each other before taking our first sips of wine/juice/water. And then we dig in, starting, of course, with a slice from the huge ham. But with my first bite, I feel the color drain from my face. I lean away from the table as the terrifying pain hits me. It's right in the middle of my chest, but I tell myself it happens right after I swallow a big bite, so it can't be a heart attack. I'm breathing fine, so I'm not choking. My thoughts are racing: what is going on?

Michelle was still a little shaken just thinking about it, as she told me her story. Her experience with an esophagus attack is familiar. I have talked to many patients who tell me a version of this story. For most people, a holiday meal focuses around a show-stopping deluxe protein. It's the same every time: ham at Easter, turkey on Thanksgiving, or prime rib at Christmas.

This tendency is so clear, it occasioned my second rule: easy solids before difficult solids. Eat easy solids to warm up your esophagus and get it better prepared for more difficult solids.

Remember our warm-ups in the last chapter? Basketball players don't walk out on the court and heave half-court shots. Football kickers don't try the sixty-yard kick at the start of their warm-up. And people prone to esophagus attacks shouldn't immediately skip from liquid to the most difficult solid. Your esophagus needs exercise before eating challenging solids. It's the second mistake I made on Curry Duck Night: not only did I go right to solids without a liquid warm-up, I also went straight to the most-likely-to-stick food—in that case, said duck.

WHAT'S AN "EASY SOLID?"

An easy solid is any solid food you *know* won't get stuck after you swallow it.

Easy solids are different for each person. Your esophagus may be wider or narrower than the next person. Corn, peas, sliced mushrooms, chopped salad, edamame, steamed green beans, and sliced cucumber are examples of foods that pass easily for most people.

WHAT'S A "DIFFICULT SOLID?"

A difficult solid is any solid food that has gotten stuck before, or that you worry will get stuck after you swallow it.

Here's a typical Sunday meal in my home. Mashed sweet potatoes, macaroni and cheese, sliced pears, and a grilled steak. A carbonated water and a glass of red wine are my liquids. I grill the steak, and I love steak, so that's what I want to eat first. It's juicy and warm. Steak is my favorite thing on the plate.

But I do not eat the warm, juicy steak first. Steak represents a difficult solid for me, as it is for many people. I sip and then gulp the water. I eat the mashed potatoes, macaroni, or a few slices of pear first. I take a sip or drink of water or wine after each solid bite (more on that in chapter 8).

So, I'll eat mashed potatoes, then macaroni and cheese, then pears. I chew and swallow at least twenty bites and evaluate. Anything stuck? After swallowing twenty easy solid bites and no issues, I cut into my steak. (More strategies for difficult solids appear in chapter 11.) I take a small bite. Chew well. Swallow. Drink a big sip or small gulp of carbonated water.

Reassess after swallowing liquid and make sure everything is clear. If in doubt, I take another drink of water.

I quietly celebrate success. When I follow my own three rules, I can enjoy the meal without an attack. Anyone who follows the system should be able to do the same.

Let's find easy solids in a variety of situations. You'll start at home. Then you'll learn restaurant strategies. You'll even eat at cocktail parties and less traditional options. You'll warm up your esophagus with easy solids and avoid difficult solids. You'll read so many options, this will be second nature. Do you know the best part? You'll warm up your esophagus, and no one will notice! With these strategies, you will gain confidence and enjoy eating with a simple scheme.

AT HOME EASY SOLIDS

Home-cooked meals are full of easy solids. Vegetables and fruit are brilliant choices. Soups always work. Well-chopped salads are staples of our meals.

Fresh corn on the cob or canned corn defines easy solid. The average kernel of corn is 0.57 inches by 0.3 inches. That's 14.5 mm by 7.6 mm if you're using the metric system. If you swallowed a whole corn kernel without chewing, it should go through your esophagus. If you struggle with corn, you must contact your healthcare provider **right away**.

Peas are another safe choice. Peas are small, 5-10 mm (0.2-0.4 inches). They are smaller than corn. You chew peas to a mushy texture. It should be easy to swallow peas and warm up your esophagus. You can't pick an easier solid than baby peas. Similar to my corn warning, if you're struggling with peas, see a doctor this week.

Mashed potatoes can be easy or difficult. It depends on consistency. Pouring potato flakes into boiling water makes thin mashed potatoes—an easy solid. The package tells you how much water to use. The flakes absorb boiling water but aren't thick. But I can make them into a problematic solid. Ever forgotten the boiling water on the stove? My three girls distract me while cooking. Sometimes, the cup of water is now two-thirds of a cup when I remember to pour in potato flakes. Poof! Distracted dad magically creates thick mashed potatoes. Swallowing thick mashed potatoes through a narrow esophagus is hard. Boiling and mashing real potatoes with butter and cream create old-fashioned mashed potatoes. Aggressively mashed potatoes are creamy—an easy solid. If chunky, they're a problematic solid. Michelle should have chosen mashed potatoes or corn before diving into her Easter ham.

Cooked vegetables make easy solids. Steamed, baked, or sautéed vegetables soften and are easier to swallow. Side dishes with potatoes, carrots, mushrooms, corn, tomatoes, green beans, and other vegetables are fine easy solids. Be careful with raw vegetables. I lost count how many times fresh carrots, celery, cauliflower, and broccoli have gotten stuck. Raw vegetables are challenging. Salad dressings and dips help. Think of salad dressings as hybrid liquids that help lubricate your esophagus. Sliced cucumber, sliced peppers, sliced mushrooms, sugar snap peas, and small tomatoes are my go-to choices on a vegetable tray. These are smaller, softer, and easier to eat. After success, I move on to raw carrots, celery, cauliflower, and broccoli.

Bananas, strawberries, blueberries, kiwi, oranges, grapefruit, pineapple, watermelon, mango, cherries, pears, raspberries, grapes, and other soft fruits are excellent choices. Soft fruits excel in warming up your esophagus. Soft fruits accompany any meal and make perfect snacks. Hard fruits, including apples, peaches, pears, nectarines, quince, and other crisp fruit that requires more chewing, are intermediate. Cut hard fruits up or chew them carefully. Harder fruits can get stuck.

Salads range from easy to tricky. Let me explain further. Aggressively chopped salads in many restaurants, Salad Creations (a salad chain), or hospitals are esophagus-friendly. Think shredded. These are easy solids. Non-chopped salads with big leaves or a tough consistency are hard for me. I struggle to eat Caesar salads with uncut romaine hearts. Spinach salads with big leaves can be challenging. Salads with big leafy greens are in between easy and difficult. Kale can be easy or difficult, depending on the variety and preparation. Kale harvested early when smaller and softer is best. Some swear by massaging kale. Google "massaging kale" and you'll find answers and methods. Avoid big-leafed or stiff kale. Kale is a healthy salad choice, but for my esophagus, it can be easy or a nightmare. Take a test bite of kale to get a sense of consistency. Wedge salads challenge my esophagus. You can still order a wedge salad at most steakhouses. Think a wedge of iceberg lettuce drizzled with salad dressing. These are difficult as a solid, and I need a fork and knife to cut it into manageable pieces.

Cottage cheese, macaroni salad, baked beans, coleslaw, and applesauce are all fantastic easy solids that are typical side dishes. They all work well to warm up my esophagus. If I don't have those choices for side dishes, I've used French fries or sweet potato fries to prepare my esophagus for more difficult solids.

This side dish list is not exhaustive. I can't begin to name them all. You get the picture. Let's discuss the next method to warm up your esophagus: appetizers!

APPETIZERS

Many terrific appetizers warm up your esophagus before a meal. Let's cover a few—but my list isn't comprehensive. Appetizers help at cocktail parties, too. As you look at appetizers and think through a warm-up strategy, focus on easy solids. Again, easy solids won't get stuck or cause an esophagus attack. Think small, easy-to-chew foods.

Soup is a perfect appetizer. A cup or small bowl of soup has ten to twenty bites to warm up your esophagus. Seafood chowders or bisques are chunky enough. You'll chew them up, but they work well. We've mentioned chopped salads, but they make a great appetizer to start a meal. If a restaurant offers to chop a salad, try it.

Chips and dip at Mexican restaurants are a winner. Miso soup, edamame, seaweed salad, and pot stickers at Japanese restaurants are all great esophagus-friendly starters. Edamame are 5-11 mm (0.2-0.43 inch) soybeans in a pod. Edamame should be an easy solid for anyone. Fresh rolls, soups, and lettuce wraps at Chinese restaurants are brilliant choices to start a meal. Various forms of cheese (cheese balls, cheese sticks, cheese dip) at bar and grill places or spinach and artichoke dip are easy solids. At Italian restaurants, start your meal with Italian soups, calamari, and various stuffed vegetables.

A cheese or charcuterie board is esophagus-friendly. Crackers, nuts, jam, honey, and other petite bites work great. Charcuterie is thin sliced meat. If the pieces are small enough, try eating the meat after fifteen to twenty successful bites. Beware of tough or thick meats. Tough meat is a precarious solid for people with esophagus problems.

Most patients tell me chicken is a challenging solid. Avoid wings as a starter. Sliders combine meat and bread—both are difficult solids. I steer away from sliders. French, Italian, and

POP QUIZ

Q. *Which one of these is NOT an easy solid?*

1. Steamed carrots.

2. Miso soup.

3. Blueberries.

4. Raw broccoli.

5. Baked beans.

Answer: 4. Raw broccoli is great for you. It's packed with nutrition. But, big hard chunks are a difficult solid.

American restaurants offer bread to begin a meal. Consider bread a challenge until your esophagus warms up. It will get stuck. The same applies to garlic bread, cheesy bread, breadsticks, or calzones. You may love chicken satay, but beware of starting a meal with chicken.

COCKTAIL PARTIES

Cocktail parties can be rough for people with a narrow esophagus. Eating sliced beef with no table and no utensils is a disaster if you have an esophageal stricture. Sometimes, I'm mid-conversation, swallow a bite, and suddenly I'm in trouble. It's frustrating and it sucks. What are some creative options? Can you avoid eating at the party? Maybe you ate before the party? Perhaps you have a meal planned afterward?

If you have a plan in place, you can choose only to consume easy solids. You can avoid chicken satay, wings, or sliced beef.

If you eat at a cocktail party, follow my three rules. To "Flush with Liquid," you need liquid, right? Water, carbonated beverages, beer, and wine all work. Once you have a liquid available, choose food carefully. Avoid problematic solids entirely.

You may not have a table to use or even utensils to cut up pieces of meat. Chapter 8 covers my third rule in detail, but here's a preview: flush every solid bite with liquid. Because this eating system uses liquid to flush things through your esophagus, you don't want to rely on alcoholic beverages unless you want to get drunk.

I hope detailed strategies at restaurants help. It equips you with the knowledge to build confidence. Release your anxiety about eating out at restaurants now. As you read through examples, focus on the simple mantra, "Easy solids before difficult solids."

AVOID THIS!

An ER doctor friend shared a story about food impactions that resonated. He explained that he hates grilling season. He said it's always the same story. Someone grills dinner outdoors. They check the meat by cutting off a piece. Maybe it's a chicken breast? Perhaps a beer bratwurst? Sometimes just a chunk of hamburger. They cut off a piece, check the internal color, and decide if it's cooked. My friend says the same thing happens every time. Rather than let that piece of meat sit, the griller eats it.

Now you know the problem. There's no warm-up—the hunk of grilled meat lodges in the esophagus. Instant esophagus attack and you meet my friend in the ER! Don't do this. You're learning how to warm up your esophagus with easy solids. In chapter 11, you'll learn a remote meat thermometer saves you from this AND helps you become a better griller.

BREAKFAST

Breakfast is less of a problem because we don't eat as much steak, chicken, pork, or ham. But you still need to stay aware, because it can happen. We cook eggs in a variety of ways, and most are an easy solid. Hard-boiled eggs are the exception and can get stuck if you aren't careful. Breakfast cereal comes in manageable pieces. Add milk, and it turns into a soft mush that's easy to swallow. Any soft fruit at breakfast is healthy and an easy solid.

Pancakes and waffles are like second cousins to bread and can be tricky unless cut into manageable pieces. Breakfast sausages are the most challenging solid at breakfast. Michelle told me they were a struggle for her, like ham. Meat for sausages is ground and encased. Be sure to warm up your esophagus and cut sausages into manageable pieces.

LUNCH

Lunch for many equals a sandwich. Meat and bread define difficult solids for many people. Should we avoid sandwiches for lunch? There are strategies for sandwiches. Make sure you have something to drink. Then look for easy solids. I can't think of a sandwich chain that doesn't sell potato chips. Chips aren't the healthiest choice, but you need something to warm up your esophagus. You can chew and swallow chips because they shatter into tiny pieces.

If you get a pickle spear, eat it before your sandwich. Old fashioned delis include a pickle because vinegar is a palate cleanser. I ignore tradition and use the pickle and chips to warm up my esophagus before I eat the sandwich. Be deliberate on your choice of bread. Less bread is better. Avoid hard, baked French bread. Choose a wrap or a tortilla. Consider your sandwich wrapped in a lettuce leaf. Try it, but beware the lettuce falling apart.

Grain bowls are a great lunch or dinner choice. These are healthy options and composed of small bites such as leafy greens, nuts, dried fruit, and cooked grains. Grain bowls often come with chicken, steak, salmon, tofu, etc. Proteins are problematic solids, so wait until you've had ten to twenty bites and your esophagus is ready. Then take a safe bite of protein and flush with liquid. More on this in chapter 8.

MUSCLE FATIGUE

Is muscular fatigue a problem while warming up your esophagus? Can I wear out my swallowing muscles? The answer is, "It's possible, but it takes a while" A study in Japan compared a group of young adults to a group of older adults with an average age of seventy-six years. They found diminished tongue pressure and diminished motor function of the lips in the older adult group after thirty minutes of eating. If the tongue and lips fatigue, they suggest other swallowing muscles fatigue. They don't limit meals to thirty minutes, but they suggest knowing that fatigue sets in if meals last longer than thirty minutes. The average mealtime was fourteen minutes for the young adults and sixteen minutes for the older adults. Unless ten to twenty small bites take you over five to ten minutes, don't worry about muscle fatigue while eating. If your mealtimes stretch out to longer than thirty minutes, muscle fatigue might be an issue. Pay attention if food tends to stick only later in meals. If this happens, esophagus muscle fatigue could be an issue.

If meals lasting thirty minutes or more cause muscle fatigue, is faster eating superior? No. As you eat and distend your stomach, hormones and neurotransmitters signal your brain that you're full. People who gorge themselves overfill their stomach before their brain says, "Stop, you're full!" Fifteen to twenty minutes is an optimal duration for your stomach, gallbladder, and pancreas to signal your brain to stop eating.

I looked for hints of esophagus attacks in history. Are we simply repeating forgotten errors? In some ways, yes. The modern-era, three-meal-a-day-diet developed in the late eighteenth century. Prior to that, humans ate two or even one large meal a day. In Terence Scully's book, *The Art of Cookery in the Middle Ages*, he notes:

> "Easily digestible foods would be consumed first, followed by gradually heavier dishes. If this regimen were not respected, it was believed that heavy foods would sink to the bottom of the stomach, thus blocking the digestion duct, so that food would digest very slowly and cause putrefaction of the body and draw bad humours into the stomach. It was also of vital importance that food of differing properties not be mixed."

Heavy foods sink to the bottom of the stomach, blocking the digestion duct? Sounds like a Middle Ages esophagus attack to me. Fascinating, right?

To summarize, eat easy solids before difficult solids, so the esophagus muscles warm up and improve coordination. You learned many methods. I'm confident you'll create your own.

Michelle refined her approach after that scary moment over

Easter lunch. Remember, she toasted the meal, so she was off to a good start (liquid before solid). But then she skipped right to what she now knows is a problematic solid. After learning the three steps, Michelle knows to warm up her esophagus to start with easy solids first, and by doing so, avoids embarrassment, uncertainty, and despair. Michelle continues to host family meals confidently, knowing she has an eating plan she can rely on, and that the simple steps will keep her esophagus issues under control.

The next chapter moves to the third and perhaps most crucial step to freeing yourself from esophagus problems and the emotional turmoil they bring with them.

CHAPTER 8

FLUSH WITH LIQUID

It was a diabetic dinner, all right: salmon and steamed vegetables. I miss dinner rolls! And steak! I know it's what's best for me, though. My doctor checked my HgA1C and it was high again (twelve). And I can't feel my toes, also not a good sign. I've got all the rules! Diabetes rules, blood pressure rules, weight loss rules. And now eating rules, too, just for swallowing! But I was doing the thing, sipping water for a warm-up, and starting out with carrots first. That was going fine for a few bites and then, bam! The pain in my chest came on strong enough, it made me curse over the dinner table with my wife.

Tim is a fifty-seven-year-old gentleman I met a few years ago. He has type 2 diabetes. HgA1C (hemoglobin A1C) measures how well Tim controls his blood sugars. Six to eight is ideal. Eight to ten means fine-tuning is in order. Over ten, like Tim's twelve, is too high. Tim knows better. Diabetes has haunted Tim for more than fifteen years. He's fifty pounds overweight. Tim suffers from high blood pressure, high cholesterol, and gastroesophageal reflux disease (GERD). Food getting stuck caused Tim to seek medical help once again. I found moderate reflux esophagitis during his esophagram. Tim actively refluxes contrast from his stomach to his throat. I give patients a 12.7 mm (1/2 inch) barium tablet during the exam (the bar test, from chapter 3). Many patients tell me it gets stuck, and I can see where it gets stuck.

The bar test helps GI doctors decide when to re-dilate their patients. When Tim swallowed the tablet, it got stuck in his distal esophagus. Curiously, though, *Tim couldn't tell*. I even had him take a couple more swallows of water. He still didn't sense the pill blockage.

For Tim, this relates to diabetes. Diabetes damages nerves—that's why he can't feel his toes.

He can't feel his esophagus either.

Tim doesn't notice the first piece of food stick because diabetes damaged the nerves. Tim has to pile up two, three, or four pieces of food before he notices it. It's much easier to get one bite of food unstuck than three.

My third rule—Flush with Liquid—applies to everyone, but it has particular significance to Tim. You must flush every solid bite with a sip or gulp of liquid.

The liquid does three critical things.

First, liquid flushes solid bites through your esophagus.

Second, liquid re-lubricates the esophagus for the next bite.

Third, liquid challenges your esophagus. Tim doesn't notice the first piece of food getting stuck. But when Tim challenges his esophagus with liquid, it flushes the solid through the narrowing. Or the stuck food alerts Tim, he drinks more liquid, and he holds off on more solid food. (Remember from chapter 6: when food obstructs, the cardinal rule is no more solid food until you've flushed with liquid until the obstruction passes.)

The Flush-With-Liquid rule saves me all the time. It helps difficult solids pass daily. It will help you, too.

When patients swallow the 12.7 mm tablet, around 30 percent of patients have trouble. But, 5-10 percent tell me the pill swallows fine, and it's blocking the distal esophagus.

If I gave them a second or third tablet, pills pile up, and the patient perceives a food blockage. Instead of piling up pills or food, a sip or gulp of liquid during the "flush with liquid" step informs you of a blockage.

"Flush each bite with liquid," might be my most critical step.

An example from medical school illustrates flush with liquid. I went to eat at a fast-food Mexican restaurant with friends. We sat down with our burritos and ate.

You can guess what happened next.

Yep, a chunk of chicken. Stuck.

In medical school, I knew some anatomy, but I was still pretty clueless. It wasn't the lightning strike of turkey at Thanksgiving; it was more of a fullness in my lower chest.

I gulped diet soda.

PAIN for about two seconds! Then instant relief.

While the emotional part of my brain was freaking out over what just happened (and I should have acknowledged that more), my analytical side realized flushing with liquid fixed the problem instantly.

In chapter 6, you learned many liquids are okay. I prefer carbonated beverages over non-carbonated beverages. Find your preferred liquid and sip or gulp it after each bite.

Consider your esophagus as a vertical pipe in your chest. When something blocks a pipe, liquid pushes at the blockage. Water adds pressure and lubricates the blockage in the tube to help it pass. The same is true for your esophagus.

Flush with liquid applies to easy solids and difficult solids. Flush every solid bite with liquid.

I waited tables at a steakhouse in Topeka, Kansas, between high school and college. Our friend Tim from this chapter would have loved this place. Many fine dining restaurants offer free bread to begin the meal. This steakhouse offered cinnamon rolls! Anyway, I saw "Flush with Liquid" in action then but didn't put it together until years later. At some tables, people ate steak and barely drank anything. Then, some customers would say at the beginning of the meal, "You might as well leave the water pitcher nearby because

I'll drink it dry." As an attentive waiter, I never did that, but I would refill their water glass eight or more times during the meal.

Looking back, the water pitcher customers probably struggled with esophagus problems and knew flushing with liquid worked.

Let's illustrate flush with liquid with another example. Imagine you're meeting friends for sushi. You might be nervous. You've read this book. The principles work at home, but you haven't tried sushi at home. Water and green tea are your liquids. You order a roll or two and ask for edamame as an appetizer. You sipped green tea and gulped water before the edamame arrives. You chew and swallow salty edamame with confidence, and you have no trouble keeping up with the conversation.

Now, the sushi arrives. Sticky rice! Chunks of fish! Does your anxiety return? Remember your strategy? You've taken liquid first. Then you enjoyed edamame and warmed up your esophagus. Start with a small bite. Chew it up and swallow. Remember to flush with liquid. Success!

How will you acknowledge success?

Enjoy the variety of flavors, the green tea, and the conversation with friends. Be grateful for your progress and triumph.

Acknowledge family and friends who have supported your journey.

If nothing else sticks from this chapter (pun intended), remember this: "Flush every bite with liquid."

That was Tim's mistake. He ate his steamed carrots but forgot to flush with liquid. Tim has medical challenges like chronic GERD, obesity, and diabetes, so he had an especially bountiful cornucopia of emotions around his health. He feels trapped by his diseases and desires. Years of porterhouse and cinnamon-roll dinners—his favorite—caught up with Tim. He's frustrated at a salmon-and-carrots diet, quickly angers when food gets stuck, and falls into despair and hopelessness.

Adding to the misfortune, from my perspective, is the fact that some changes ten or twenty years ago could have avoided esophagus attacks today. Read on to chapter 9 and learn what you can do to keep a minimal esophagus problem from getting worse.

PART 3

MANAGING YOUR ESOPHAGUS

CHAPTER 9

LIFESTYLE CHANGES

It took Zoey a minute to remember what she'd been prescribed before for GERD, but finally she got it: Omeprazole. One pill half an hour before breakfast, she remembered. But she also remembered it didn't work. Took it a couple of times, to deal with the weird taste in her mouth and the pain in her chest, but nothing really changed. So she stopped taking it.

The GERD didn't stop, though. It does seem better; she only has burning once or twice a week now—better than the every night experience when she was pregnant! Anyway, it can't be that big a deal, she figured, all those commercials on TV must mean it is really common. Why worry?

Zoey knew if she went to the doctor, she was just going to hear, again, about stopping smoking and losing weight. Like it was that easy. She guessed she'd just deal with the burning now and then.

Many patients like Zoey are confused about GERD and its treatment. So I want to clear some things up. This chapter will focus on how to treat reflux without pills—the medication options will follow in the next chapter. Either way, it's equally important to find relief for your symptoms now, and keep a slight problem from getting worse.

QUICK REVIEW FROM CHAPTER 2

To make sure you're ready to make sense of the advice in this chapter, take a moment to refresh yourself on information from chapter 2. Gastroesophageal reflux (GER) occurs when stomach acid flows upward to the esophagus. Gastroesophageal reflux disease (GERD) is the same as GER, but it causes pain or another problem.

Occasional reflux (GER) is normal after eating. These episodes are painless and brief.

Patients with GERD often complain of dull, burning chest pain that's worse when they lie down. Chronic untreated GERD causes changes in the esophagus over the years to decades. Chronic changes can narrow the esophagus (i.e., stricture) and even, rarely, cause esophageal cancer.

ZOEY'S FEARS

Zoey lives in a kind of denial—not about GERD; she knows

she has that—but about the fact that smoking, obesity, and GERD are real problems for her, problems that she *could* do something about. The multiple questions about GERD still buzzing around her mind signal to me that she's open to learning more and taking action if I can convince her it will make a difference.

Zoey projects her frustration onto her doctor, imagining what she will say (and won't be able to do). And she may be right—some physicians may struggle to empathize with patients dealing with issues they haven't experienced themselves. Still, Zoey needed to know more about the lifestyle changes, over-the-counter medications, and prescription medications she could use as tools to fix GERD.

Healthcare gets more expensive each year, yet physicians see more patients and burn out. Physicians discussed the strengths and weaknesses of lifestyle choices years ago—times change. Physicians click a mouse, and your prescription is ready for pick-up fifteen minutes later at your pharmacy. It is the Amazon-ification of medicine. Physician time constraints mean cutting corners, and lifestyle choice discussions got cut out of GERD appointments decades ago.

If you want to skip ahead to pill-based solutions, they are ahead in chapter 10. Pill-based solutions to GERD are temporary solutions to an ongoing problem. If you continue smoking, eating fast-food late at night, and continue to gain excess weight, the pill-based solutions will help for a few months. Maybe years. But you will re-injure your esophagus.

CANCER

The elephant in the room is cancer. Every time I perform an esophagram, the first thing I talk about is whether I think my patient has cancer. Remember, back to chapter 1: 99 percent of you with esophagus attacks don't have cancer. One percent will have cancer. Chronic reflux damages the esophagus and transforms the esophagus cells into stomach cells. Chapter 2 briefly covered this, and we dive deeper in chapter 12. We call this transformation Barrett's esophagus. Injured cells, over years or decades, rarely turn into esophageal cancer. Think of reflux like sun exposure or smoking.

Smoke enough cigarettes long enough, and your chances of lung cancer keep going up. Spending too much time in the sun damages the skin and causes skin cancer. Chronic acid reflux into your esophagus causes injury and rarely causes cancer.

GENETICS?

Is there a genetic basis for GERD or esophageal cancer? The best answer is: we don't know. Researchers have tested specific genes, but they have discovered no direct link. There are more than twenty spots in our genetic code that if something's wrong, it increases your risk for esophageal cancer, but there's no direct link.

LIFESTYLE MODIFICATIONS

Simple changes you make that reduce reflux are lifestyle modifications. I divide these simple changes into three levels. The first level is feasible and easy. You should be aware of second-level changes, but they have less impact or are more challenging. The third level changes are essential but hard to attain. It's easier to climb a 200-foot hill than a 13,000-foot peak in Colorado. I'll tell you about the 200-foot hills you can conquer and discuss the mountain climbs later.

Most guides to GERD say lose weight, stop smoking, and eat a better diet.

Lose weight? HARD!

Stop smoking? HARDER!

Eat a better diet? What's that? There are over 500 diets. What's a better diet?

This chapter gives you achievable stepping stones that lead toward achieving harder changes.

FIRST LEVEL LIFESTYLE MODIFICATIONS
FOUR-HOUR RULE

GER is stomach contents moving to your esophagus. If I never lay down, I'll never have reflux, right? There's truth here. We know from pH probe studies humans can reflux upright, but it's rare. We also know people reflux more lying down or asleep. What if you could reduce reflux by 80 percent or 90 percent by avoiding eating four hours before bedtime? Achievable? Attainable? Realistic? I'm a physician with young children, and I made this change. Knowledge is power—power over your fear and anxiety. You can make a positive change.

If you plan to sleep at ten o'clock in the evening, finish eating by six o'clock. Before you say, "That's too hard," think about it. You can make it work. Shift caloric intake earlier in the day. As adults, we don't need 1,000 or more calories in the evening. You don't need a large meal to sleep overnight. You're busy at work, or you may have late meetings. You may not get home until after seven o'clock or eight o'clock in the evening. Eat a small dinner or skip the evening meal. When you wake, you'll be hungry. You may even go to sleep with a grumbling belly. On those evenings with little or no food, you can relax about GERD because there's almost no chance you're refluxing overnight. There is active research investigating fasting and changing meal times to lose weight. I'm not writing a diet book, but eating less at your last meal may help you lose weight.

If you have diabetes and need to maintain a specific blood sugar, ask your doctor or your dietician how to shift calories earlier in the day.

A trial illustrated the four-hour rule. Doctors performed endoscopy to look for reflux before the trial. Then they placed a pH probe in the esophagus to measure reflux episodes. In the study, patients ate dinner at either five o'clock in the evening or nine o'clock, then went to bed at eleven o'clock. I nicknamed this the McDonald's trial because patients received meal vouchers at McDonald's for a Big Mac, medium fries, and a medium drink. No surprise, patients reflux more when they ate the nine o'clock meal and less from the five o'clock meal. If the patient was overweight, reflux was much worse. Patients with esophagitis or a hiatal hernia had even more reflux from the nine o'clock meal. Esophagitis is irritation of the esophagus. In chapter 2, you learned a hiatal hernia occurs when part of your stomach moves into the chest and worsens reflux. The McDonald's trial says if you eat dinner and lie down to sleep two hours later, you suffer more GERD. Simple solution: move your last meal earlier in the day. Or skip it.

Another study confirmed the McDonald's trial. Twenty-three healthy volunteers monitored esophagus pH levels to assess for reflux. They had standard meals for breakfast, lunch, and then either an early six o'clock in the evening dinner or a late nine o'clock in the evening dinner. Which group had more reflux? You guessed it; the nine o'clock group! The McDonald's trial applied to patients with esophagus problems and obesity. This trial proved healthy people reflux overnight if they eat a late dinner.

What if you take a nap? The same thinking applies. If you lie down with a full stomach, reflux worsens. Try to give yourself four hours. If you plan on a nap, limit caloric intake at your midday meal.

If you're on the fence about a smaller evening meal or waiting four hours, let's talk more about sleep and the last meal of the day. Sleep isn't my medical specialty, but let's go over some basics. Your body continues functioning while you sleep, so you're still burning calories. Many Americans eat more calories during their last meal of the day than they need to sleep. The equation is 0.42 x bodyweight in pounds x hours of sleep. For me, that's 0.42 x 160 pounds x 8 hours = 538 calories. You don't need a large dinner to sustain your energy needs overnight. I only need 538 calories.

Your body stores up around 2,000 calories in your liver and muscles. You don't need an enormous meal before sleep—it worsens reflux.

Does GER impact sleep? Yes! If you struggle with sleep, you're not alone. Of 1,000 people with GERD, 79 percent reported nighttime heartburn, and 75 percent of these people felt it affected their sleep. Forty percent believed it altered their daytime functioning. Another study shows sleep-related GER decreases sleep quality, increases arousals from rest, causes more fatigue, and decreases work productivity. Does any of this sound like you?

A trial tested this data. Seven hundred and fifty people with sleep-related GERD received either a full-strength PPI, a half-strength PPI, or a placebo for six weeks. The patients who received the PPI reported better sleep, better work productivity, and gained back lost work hours.

A large survey of 11,685 Americans reached the same conclusions. Patients with reflux and sleep difficulty had more healthcare visits, a 5.5 percent loss of work productivity, and reduced quality of life.

Zoey was dubious about this change, but when she realized eating an earlier and smaller meal reduced reflux, improved her sleep, and helped her GERD, she was all-in. Triple-wins are hard to find.

Is a PPI a sleep aid? No! Don't take a pill if changing your last meal time fixes the problem. If you keep four hours between your last meal and bedtime, you won't reflux as much, and you might even sleep better. If you suffer from GERD, ask yourself if you can eat a smaller dinner or skip dinner. You might even lose weight. Win-win. This book isn't about diet or sleep, but knowing more will help you make the best decision.

NO TIGHT CLOTHES TO SLEEP

Skintight clothes cause reflux. Imagine you skip the four-hour rule. You ate dinner at nine o'clock in the evening and lay down at ten o'clock. You likely reflux your dinner into your esophagus overnight.

How do we know? Several studies have shown as a patient's waist circumference and body mass index go up, there is higher pressure in the stomach. One study put weight lifter's belts on patients with known GERD and esophagus injury. They measured the pressure in the stomach with no weight belt and then with a weight belt applied. They counted reflux events with no weight belt and with a weight belt. No surprise—the pressure in the stomach is higher with the weight belt applied. Gastroesophageal reflux increased eight-fold with the weight belt around their belly.

The pressure the weight belt applies to the abdomen is the same as tight-fitting clothes. The most obvious example is Spanx shapewear. Nothing against this brand, but avoid sleeping in tight-fitting clothes over your abdomen if you suffer from reflux. Wear tight-fitting clothes when you don't worry about reflux. Wear it to work, dinner, routine activities, or exercise. Avoid it while sleeping.

AVOID THE THREE F'S

I tell my patients with reflux to avoid the three Fs: fast, fried, and fatty foods worsen reflux.

How do we know? A 2018 study measured the esophagus and stomach acid levels after three unique meals. Researchers prepared meals with equal calories and equal volume but different percentages of fat, carbohydrate, and protein. There was a high-fat meal, a standard meal, and a functional food meal. They gave these three meals in distinct orders over twenty-six hours, including pH monitoring overnight. They studied three patient groups. Group 1 patients had reflux esophagitis (RE) and complained of heartburn symptoms. These patients had mild proven esophagus damage. Group 2 patients had non-erosive reflux disease (NERD). These patients complained of heartburn symptoms but didn't have esophagus damage. Group 3 patients were healthy, with no complaints and a normal esophagus. After the high-fat meal, the patients with RE and NERD had higher acid levels in their esophagus. Acid levels peaked two hours after eating and remained elevated at three hours. It returned to the same level as the other meals at four hours.

Why? Foods with a higher fat content take longer to digest. Higher fat content foods slow down your GI tract. Food sits in your stomach and proximal bowel longer. Because food sits longer, there's a greater chance for reflux. I'm not saying no to fast, fried, or fatty—all things in moderation.

You should avoid a fried, fatty, fast-food meal late at night if you suffer from reflux. Eat a healthy choice if it's late or skip it.

Allow four hours from when you eat solid food until you lie down. Knowing higher fat content foods take longer to digest, you will make better lifestyle changes and reduce reflux.

My first GERD episode burns in my memory. Yours may, too. I broke all my own rules before I knew any rules or thought of creating them. Imagine a third-year medical student enjoying a Kansas City Royals baseball game just after seven o'clock in the evening. I did everything wrong. I wolfed down a foot-long hot dog, chili cheese fries, and a beer around eight o'clock in the evening. Dessert came during the eighth inning—ice cream, whipped cream, and a deep-fat-fried cone. I ate this closer to ten o'clock in the evening. Around eleven o'clock, I returned to my apartment and went to sleep.

Around half past midnight, I woke with a start. I vividly remember two things. There was an awful burning chest pain. Not the burning embers Lauren describes in chapter 2. The burning deep in my chest was closer to a backyard bonfire after you add newspaper. I had a feeling of impending doom, dark and foreboding, like a thunderstorm rolling in and turning daylight to darkness. Third-year medical students know enough to be dangerous, so my first thought with chest pain and impending doom was a heart attack. As I shook the daze of sleep from my brain, I reminded myself I'm in my twenties, I woke from sleep, and I'm otherwise healthy. I realized there was zero chance of a heart attack. The next thought was GERD. Everything I'd eaten in the previous four hours was fast, fried, and fatty. My ten o'clock in the evening waffle cone sundae tasted great but took revenge on my foolish youth.

Four antacid tablets snuffed out the flickering flames in my chest. Five minutes later, the thunderstorm of doom passed. I felt reborn while I deeply exhaled, closed my eyes, and dropped back into sleep. But I knew I had GERD.

If you've experienced this, it's okay. You're reading this book and learning more about GERD. Keep reading to learn how to reduce reflux or avoid it.

EXERCISE

You should exercise. Some people perceive painless reflux during exercise. I sometimes do. Should I worry? Nope, no pain. Exercise *reduces* GERD and the risk of esophageal cancer. This makes sense. Exercise may occasionally induce reflux, but don't worry about it. Healthy people can have occasional reflux. The positives of exercise outweigh the negatives of occasional reflux. You'll learn more about obesity being a powerful risk factor for GERD. Exercise is key to reducing our obesity epidemic.

CHEW GUM

Chewing gum stimulates the salivary glands in the mouth and creates more saliva. Chewing gum increases salivary flow rates, bicarbonate in saliva, and also makes you swallow. The bigger the gum, the higher the increase in salivary flow.

Saliva is basic, so it neutralizes gastric acid in the distal esophagus and washes it back into your stomach.

In short, chewing sugar-free gum is an excellent way to reduce reflux.

Let's transition from the first level of no-brainer changes to reduce GERD to the second level. The second level is potential changes you should be aware of but have less impact or are more challenging to achieve. These suggestions help you gain knowledge and power over fears or misconceptions about GERD.

SECOND LEVEL LIFESTYLE CHANGES
EAT CLEAN

Some eat food for pleasure. Some consider food as fuel. If you struggle with GERD, I invite you to think of food as healing medicine. Whole, unprocessed, natural food is some of the best functional medicine you can put in your body for many reasons. The prime reason I recommend it to my patients, though, is that it helps heal GERD.

For more GERD-specific information on clean eating, I recommend *The Acid Watcher Diet* by ENT Dr. Jonathan Aviv, which adds an anti-reflux focus to general clean-eating principles.

If you are a social media user, you might want to look for like-minded clean eaters using the #FoodIsFuel and #Eat-Clean hashtags.

CHOCOLATE

Too often, patients associate lifestyle modification as completely giving up something they love. I love chocolate. Chocolate causes reflux. It has methylxanthine, which reduces the lower esophageal sphincter pressure, causing the sphincter to contract less, causing reflux. Will I give up chocolate? No way. Will I eat a slice of chocolate cheesecake an hour before bedtime? No way. Small amounts of chocolate earlier in the day are fine, but skip it four hours before you sleep.

MINT

Another favorite flavor of mine is mint. Peppermint and spearmint are carminatives, which are oil extracts from plants. Medical literature says avoid mint if you have reflux or GERD. A study put this to the test. They gave mint to groups of people to see if mint increased reflux. It didn't. I haven't given up mint, and you don't have to either. That said, something like Lauren's chocolate mint milkshake, from chapter 2, a couple of hours before bedtime isn't a great idea.

COFFEE

Another thing I love is coffee, so I wasn't eager to give this up, either. If you Google "causes of reflux," you will find coffee on the list. There is controversy, though, in the medical literature about whether coffee causes reflux. You can find evidence on both sides. A large meta-analysis concluded there was no significant contribution to reflux by coffee. Two more large trials found no relationship between coffee drinking and GERD. So if you have reflux, don't worry about coffee unless you notice a specific negative effect in your body.

CARBONATED BEVERAGES

Do carbonated beverages cause reflux? Let's return to your chemistry class for a minute and remember the pH scale. A liquid's pH is how acidic or basic and ranges from 1-14.

Let's start right in the middle of the pH scale. Distilled water is neutral with a pH of 7.0. Any number smaller than 7.0 is acidic, and any number bigger than 7.0 is basic. The pH of the gastric acid in your stomach ranges from 1.5 to 3.5. Sodas like Pepsi (2.39), Coke (2.5), and Sprite (3.29) have low pH values. Citrus drinks like orange juice (pH 3.3-4.2), grapefruit juice (pH 3.8), cranberry juice (2.5), and tomato juice (pH 4.1-4.6) have low pH values, too. Most beers have a pH of around 4.0, and most wines have a pH of 3.0-4.0.

Less acidic options include carbonated mineral waters like Perrier, Eska, Pelligrino, and Gerolsteiner, with pH values of 5.3-6. And, backing up what I said about coffee above, Starbucks' medium roast coffee has a pH of 5.11. If you like your coffee light, know that the pH of skim milk is 6.8.

A medical survey connected carbonated beverages with GERD. That's a survey, and it didn't test patients with pH monitors or have them drink water, then Coke, and vice versa. Don't change your behavior based on a medical survey. Carbonated beverages have a low pH. Try to drink ones that have better pH values. I drink carbonated beverages but avoid them four hours before bedtime.

FIBER

Generally speaking, getting more fiber in your diet is helpful in cases of GERD. Natural sources of fiber may reduce reflux, and help you lose weight, as well as improve bowel regularity. As with anything else, you don't want to go overboard.

Dietary fiber and GERD are controversial. Physicians always quibble about research articles, and there are weaknesses in the article I'm about to tell you about, but it is interesting nonetheless: a small study compared fiber to an over-the-counter reflux medication (Ranitidine 75 mg twice daily) to placebo (four starch capsules) over two weeks. Fiber decreased heartburn severity, similar to the drug.

ALCOHOL

Ever been to a party where you're the sober person, and everyone else is intoxicated? Did you see impaired coordination? Yes. Muscles that don't contract well? Yep. Inhibitions reduced? Uh-huh. Since your esophagus is primarily a muscular tube, it's stumbling around. It has lost its coordination, like the intoxicated person.

When you drink alcohol, it affects your esophagus. Your stomach secretes more acid. Your lower esophageal sphincter relaxes, which allows more reflux. It impairs the muscular contraction patterns and coordination of the esophagus. In other words, alcohol messes with your esophagus.

Alcohol and GERD stimulate arguments between doctors. There are more trials about alcohol and GERD than about chocolate, spicy foods, citrus drinks, carbonated beverages, mint, and late evening meals put together. On balance, these studies suggest more reflux symptoms and GERD in modest or heavy alcohol users than non-drinkers.

Similar to chocolate and mint, be aware of this information and make an informed decision. In medical school, I might have downed a Big Mac and fries with a glass of merlot. Today, I enjoy a restaurant cheeseburger and glass of red wine at least four hours before bedtime.

SPICY FOODS

Many patients tell me spicy foods cause reflux. "Spicy foods GERD" returns 510,000 results on Google with the top ten results strongly favoring a connection. There's little actual medical evidence linking spicy foods and GERD, however.

One suggestive piece is the 1990 study in which thirty-two people took part in a small trial. Half were healthy, and half had a history of heartburn. All had a pH probe placed, which detects acid in the esophagus.

On day one, all participants had a plain hamburger and a glass of water. The following day, they had the same hamburger and water, but added a slice of onion to the hamburger. In the healthy patients, no reflux occurred. In patients with a history of heartburn, the onion slice caused significant reflux.

Researchers concluded onions are "a potent and long-lasting refluxogenic agent" in heartburn patients. In other words, the spicy foods caused reflux in patients with reflux.

While I may have some doubts about the onion article, mostly because of its small size—and, how spicy is an onion, anyway?—a more recent Korean research adds validity. This study, though, didn't confirm reflux with a pH probe. Korean researchers surveyed one hundred twenty-six patients. Doctors suspected all had a history of reflux. They studied all patients with upper endoscopy and pH monitoring, then divided into two groups. Group 1 had proven GERD. Group 2 possibly had GERD based on testing. All patients completed surveys about one hundred fifty-two foods asking about reflux symptoms. Hot spicy stews, rice cakes, ramen noodles, fried foods, and topokki scored highest for causing reflux.

My conclusion on spicy foods?

All things in moderation. If you love and crave spicy foods, be curious about and aware of your symptoms afterward. Empower yourself to be an experimental lab and try out ideas. Don't eat hot spicy Korean stew and lie down for bed an hour later!

CITRUS

Seventy-two percent of four hundred surveyed GERD patients said citrus fruits cause heartburn. Stop eating oranges? No. When physicians test this on patients, they don't reproduce it. I don't limit citrus fruits or juices.

Do you feel more knowledgeable about the foods cited for causing gastroesophageal reflux?

You should. Have a plan? It could be:

1. I'll keep enjoying my peppermint mocha lattes in the morning as long as it doesn't bother my reflux.

Or

2. I'll eat a smaller meal at seven o'clock each night, since I lay down at nine o'clock.

Once you know details, you can make wise choices. Wise choices allow positive gains over GERD and your fears.

THIRD LEVEL LIFESTYLE CHANGES

The third level of lifestyle changes is hard. You should know them and they may help you. Some may not work for everyone (head of bed elevation), or they're tough to achieve (weight loss).

SLEEP ON AN ANGLE

Physicians educate patients with reflux to elevate the head of their bed. When I was in medical school more than twenty years ago, a physician told his patient to do this. The patient and I both had a confused look on our faces. The physician instructed the patient to raise the head of the bed with bricks or concrete blocks. They recommended five to twenty degrees. Let's hope the bed never slipped off the bricks or blocks!

The proper question: Does sleeping on an angle help? Several studies say yes. So try it?

Before you put bricks or cinder blocks under your bed posts, there are better solutions. Angled body pillows cost $50-$100 on Amazon.

An adjustable bed is more expensive, but if the angled pillow helps you, this might be more accessible.

Good adjustable beds cost $1,500-$3,000.

Recliners work for a night or two, but not long-term.

Here's the rub. Sleeping on an angle is hard on your body. When you sleep flat, your weight distributes over your entire body. When you sleep in a recliner or on an angled pillow, your body weight centers to your butt and legs. Blood may pool in your legs, and leg swelling develops. Pressure points form and may cause pain.

Sleeping positioned to stop reflux might help. Sleeping flat on your back worsens reflux. Especially with a full belly. Right-side-down sleeping moves fluid away from the esophagus. Belly sleeping works the same, but not as well. Beware—neither helps back pain. Many people move while they sleep. Focusing efforts on sleeping in a particular position may fail.

Before you buy an angle pillow or an expensive adjustable bed, try to solve the problem yourself. Avoid eating late in the evening. Try to fix your actual problem before compensating with something else.

STOP SMOKING

If you smoke, do all you can to stop. Many physicians, myself included, have never smoked. I only know secondhand the immense challenge of quitting.

Cigarettes and nicotine are addictive and difficult to quit. You will need guidance from a physician, an addiction specialist, a counselor, and countless others to stop. If you're a smoker, please get help. Zoey, from earlier in this chapter, knew she needed to stop smoking but didn't realize the tight link between smoking and GERD.

Cigarette smoking worsens gastroesophageal reflux in three ways. Smoking relaxes muscles, including the lower esophageal sphincter (LES). When the LES relaxes, reflux occurs. When you smoke, you make less saliva. Saliva is mostly water but has bicarbonate. Swallowing saliva neutralizes acid in the esophagus and clears acid from your esophagus. Less saliva means less acid removed from the esophagus. Smoking increases reflux episodes compared with nonsmokers.

Want more marvelous news about quitting cigarette smoking? Quitting helps GERD. Smokers with GERD who stopped noticed their GERD severity scores improved.

NEVER VAPE

We don't know the relationship between vaping (e-cigarettes) and GERD. But vaping nicotine should lower distal esophageal sphincter pressure and increase reflux. Vaping is harmful for a variety of other reasons. If you vape, try to stop. If you don't vape, don't start. Don't use vaping to quit smoking unless your physician endorses it.

OBESITY

If I could snap my fingers and my patients would lose weight, that would reduce GERD. Obesity is a national epidemic, and losing weight is hard. I see the consequences of obesity daily. Higher body mass index (BMI) causes more GERD symptoms. I've struggled to lose weight. Members of my family and friends struggle with it. Searching for "weight-loss book" on Amazon returns upwards of 90,000 results!

Lose weight by making better lifestyle choices. Don't eat late at night. If you can't eat dinner before seven o'clock in the evening, eat a small dinner like a high protein yogurt or a protein bar and stop. Don't eat fast food. Exercise more. With simple changes, you can improve GERD and enjoy weight loss success. It helps me, and I hope it helps you.

CHANGES WORK

Let's revisit Zoey and look at the changes she ultimately

decided to take after learning that experiencing chest pain after eating, even one or two days a week, was definitely *not* normal—and *is* avoidable.

The first change that worked was to see a new doctor, one who Zoey felt listened to her and understood her. (Even if the subjects of smoking and weight still came up.)

The doctor recommended the same medication Zoey had tried before but insisted Zoey take it every day for two months, no matter how she felt, before she decided if it was helpful. The pain slowly improved each day for a week, then went away altogether.

The long-term solution, though, to avoid relying on medicine forever, was when Zoey changed how she ate. *Not* as in dieting, though some weight loss did occur, but as in *scheduling*. The important part was that Zoey stopped eating big meals at night. She ate a big breakfast, but a small dinner.

These simple initial changes catapulted Zoey into a cascade of better choices. Zoey's sleep improved because she had less nocturnal GERD. She woke up rested and energized. She found exercise in the morning appealed to her now. She got more steps each day and lost about ten pounds. Her GERD abated, and so did her denial, frustration, and uncertainty about her health.

Zoey's experience shows that PPIs and H-2 blockers (medications described in the next chapter) decrease stomach acid so the esophagus can heal, but they aren't always a complete solution all by themselves. When you stop the pill, you risk GERD returning if nothing else changes.

The lifestyle changes Zoey made, though, eliminated her need for medication—after the two months, she stopped taking it and found that her other changes were now enough to keep the GERD under control. A month later, still no pain! She understands, though, that medication can work for her if she needs it. And for readers in a similar situation, chapter 10 explains pill-based treatments for GERD.

CHAPTER 10

MEDICATIONS

It's getting tight again, Doc. Chicken and beef get stuck if I'm not careful. I stopped Omeprazole, but I get heartburn in a few weeks, and my stricture gets tighter faster. After the last balloon dilation, I went to 10 mg Omeprazole every other day. That seems to work, but steak triggers me. It's been eighteen months since my last dilation—no problem with easy solids. Liquids are no problem. But, you know, I love my steak!

Jim joined the Marines long enough ago that he fought for his country in the Korean War, and he has battled GERD just about as long. He has had GERD since his twenties, when he developed a hiatal hernia. He's dealt with a tight esophagus since his forties. He started on Ranitidine back in the early 1980s and switched to Omeprazole in the early 1990s.

Still, his mild esophagus stricture is a daily challenge, and his gastroenterologist dilates Jim's esophagus a few times each decade. On the plus side, Jim's never had surgery, Barrett's esophagus, or cancer.

Ever had a sunburn? Too much sunlight injured your skin, it turned pink or red, and it hurt. GERD is like the sunburn. Too much acid exposure causes the esophagus to turn pink or red and hurts. These medicines decrease stomach acid. Less acid means your esophagus can heal, like your skin healing the sunburn. You can do many things to decrease sun exposure: cover up, use a sun umbrella, stay inside, or apply sunblock. For reflux, lifestyle choices (eat clean, allow four hours before lying down, etc.) are the best choice. But medications speed healing and protect from acid injury.

Let's learn more about pill-based solutions to stop GERD and heal your esophagus.

PROTON PUMP INHIBITORS (PPIS)

DRUG NAME	COMMON COMMERCIAL NAME(S)	OTC/RX
ESOMEPRAZOLE	Nexium	Both
LANSOPRAZOLE	Prevacid	Both
OMEPRAZOLE	Prilosec	Both
PANTOPRAZOLE	Protonix	Both
RABEPRAZOLE	AcipHex	Rx only

Proton pump inhibitors (PPIs) are the best medications for GERD. They block an acid pump in your stomach for thirty-six to ninety-six hours, so you take them once daily. Patients are more likely to remember medicines that are once-daily rather than twice or three times daily. Take it thirty minutes before your first meal. Some patients need PPIs twice daily for acid suppression and healing. If prescribed twice daily, take it thirty minutes before breakfast and thirty minutes before dinner.

PPIs inhibit stomach acid production. Because there's less acid, the esophagus can heal. PPIs heal 84-95 percent of erosive esophagitis after eight weeks of daily treatment. Those are phenomenal healing rates. We'll talk about H2 blockers, but they have a 70-77 percent success rate in healing esophagitis.

Ever broken a bone? To heal a bone, doctors immobilize it in a cast. The cast holds the bones in alignment, and your bones heal. You keep a cast on for four to six weeks. Your body has a remarkable ability to heal itself. The same idea applies to PPI medicines to heal your esophagus. Take your PPI for thirty or sixty days. Stopping a PPI after a few days is like ripping off the cast three days after applying it. You can't see bones heal, and you can't see your esophagus heal. Don't rip off the cast, and don't stop the PPI.

Take the medication as your doctor directs—thirty days minimum and up to sixty days for others.

Let's say you only take the PPI when you have the pain or reflux symptoms. I've heard this before. Would you cast a broken bone one day and take it off the next day? Many patients tell me they only take their PPI when they have symptoms, and it doesn't help them. It only helps if you take it thirty or sixty days as directed by your doctor to help your body heal.

People often ask, "What do I do after thirty or sixty days?" Follow your doctor's advice. You stop the PPI and your doctor presumes your esophagus healed. Your healthcare provider hopes your lifestyle changes prevent GERD relapse. We call this approach step-down therapy. After one year, 58 percent of patients relapse and go back on a PPI. If this happens, discuss options with your doctor. They may recommend fourteen or thirty days of daily PPI therapy to get you healed again. If GERD returns, consider maintenance therapy. This is a reduced dose of PPI. One choice is half your treatment dose daily. For example, if you take 20 mg Omeprazole daily for therapy, the maintenance dose is 10 mg daily. Another choice is to take the PPI at your regular dose every other day. In other words, if you were on 20 mg Omeprazole daily to heal the esophagus, you'd take 20 mg Omeprazole every other day for maintenance. Jim, the former Marine from earlier in the chapter, worked on step-down therapy with his doctor to reduce his Omeprazole.

What if you've taken your PPI religiously and you're still having pain? Your first PPI prescription may not heal your esophagus. Don't despair, step out of your fear cave, and tell your doctor. They may increase your dose. Many studies show superior healing with a higher dose.

Your doctor will have options for you. Including:

Add an H2 blocker.

Increase your PPI to twice daily.

Take the PPI to twice daily plus add an H2 blocker.

Doctors try to treat you with as few pills as possible.

A rare, hard-to-treat type of GERD is gaining recognition called nocturnal GERD. Some patients taking a PPI twice a day still have acid break-through overnight sometime between ten o'clock in the evening and six o'clock in the morning. This breakthrough GERD happens when you're asleep. You probably don't know it. The only sign might be a random overnight wake-up. Ever wake up at night for no apparent reason and have a funny taste in your mouth? Some call it "gastric acid recovery" because the acidity of the stomach recovers overnight despite suppression. If your physician suspects you have nocturnal or break-through GERD, the best approach is to adjust your PPI dosing schedule. They may also add an H2 blocker before bedtime.

TYPICAL APPROACH TO INCREASING DOSE FOR UNCONTROLLED GERD

PPI once a day
PPI plus H2 blocker
PPI twice a day
PPI twice a day plus H2 blocker

Doctors have over thirty years of experience with PPIs since Omeprazole came out in 1990. These medications have an excellent safety profile. There is a potential risk of colon infection or a lung infection like pneumonia while taking a PPI. The strong acid secreted by our stomach kills bacteria and fungi. When stomach acid decreases, it may not kill as many bacteria.

There is conflicting data about long-term use of PPIs and bone density. Long-term is not thirty or sixty days–long-term is years. Two studies tested long-term or high dose PPI therapy and found some evidence of bone loss. Some suggest if you need long-term or high dose PPI therapy to increase your dietary calcium intake. Milk, cheese, yogurt, sardines, salmon, and seeds increase dietary calcium. Supplemental calcium (aka calcium pills) is another option. I have zero concern about bone loss from sixty days on a PPI. Six months or a year catches my eye. Three or six years makes me think hard about calcium supplementation.

Don't lose sleep about the low risks of issues with PPIs. Do everything in your power to make lifestyle changes so you don't need to rely on PPIs to stop GERD.

H-2 BLOCKERS

Histamine-2 receptor antagonists (H-2 blockers) block acid production like PPIs. H-2 blockers work, but PPIs work better. PPIs achieve 84-95 percent healing, and H-2 blockers achieve 70-77 percent healing. Higher doses result in better healing rates. Why even consider a second-class medicine? H-2 blockers cost less. A thirty-day supply of an H2 blocker averages $20. A thirty-day supply of an over-the-counter PPI is $60, and a prescription supply might cost $200.

DRUG NAME	COMMON COMMERCIAL NAME	OTC/RX
Cimetidine	Tagamet	Both
Famotidine	Pepcid or Pepcid AC	Both
Nizatidine	Axid or Tazac	Both
Ranitidine	Zantac	Both

Don't take H-2 blockers and antacids together. Tums and Rolaids stop your stomach from absorbing an H-2 blocker.

OVER-THE-COUNTER MEDICATIONS

Tums and Rolaids are over the counter chewable pills that contain basic ingredients like calcium carbonate that neutralize acid. Gaviscon is a similar medication that contains magnesium and aluminum to neutralize gastric acid. I took Tums when post-baseball game GERD woke me from sleep, and my pain stopped. These medicines briefly help reflux symptoms but do nothing to heal the esophagus injury.

As a medical student, I didn't know better. I cannot endorse these medications to treat GERD. PPIs and H-2 blockers are much better to heal the esophagus injury. If you insist on Tums or Rolaids, Walgreens makes a pill that combines 800 mg calcium carbonate (active ingredient in Tums) and 20 mg Omeprazole (a PPI).

OVER THE COUNTER OR PRESCRIPTION?

Are PPIs or H2 Blockers over-the-counter (OTC) as good as prescription (Rx) medicines? What's the difference?

The US Food and Drug Administration (FDA) states you can only take a PPI for fourteen days to reduce stomach acid.

The OTC and Rx versions are identical.

Can't I just buy the OTC version?

Prescription Omeprazole might be cheaper than buying the OTC version if you have a generous pharmacy benefit. $5 co-pay for Rx or $60 for OTC? I choose Rx every day.

Let's say your pharmacy benefit is stingy. Or you haven't met a deductible. Maybe it's $200 for the Rx version or $60 for OTC.

What to do?

My best advice: follow your doctor's advice. But know you have options and most doctors want their patients to take the medicines they prescribe. Even if sometimes it means buying them through non-traditional means.

CARAFATE

Another medication for GERD is Sucralfate, also known as Carafate. Sucralfate binds to a stomach injury, creates a physical barrier, and protects the stomach from damaging acid. We presume it does the same thing in the esophagus. Carafate doesn't heal like PPIs or H-2 blockers. So why bring it up? It is considered safer during pregnancy because your stomach and bowel don't absorb it. This medication causes constipation in 2 percent of the patients who take it. If you're prone to constipation, be aware. Consider adding more fluids to your daily intake or consider adding more fiber to compensate.

CHOOSE YOUR CHANGES

From this chapter, you know PPIs are the best medication to heal injuries to the esophagus and stomach from GERD. Lifestyle changes and medications together cure GERD. Pills heal the injury, but your lifestyle changes stop GERD from coming back. Choose from many options or combine changes for greater impact.

The most crucial thing in this chapter is the former Marine Jim's story. In partnership with his doctors, he's navigated a problematic disease with the same "can-do" attitude that's helped him throughout his life in all kinds of circumstances. As a result, he's thrived despite esophagus challenges. Because he's stayed on top of his condition, Jim eats the food he wants and lives with only mild problems with difficult foods—even at ninety.

You have a "can-do" attitude within you, too. Tap into that. Work to understand your esophagus problem. Take care of it. Physicians, mid-level providers, nurses, therapists, technologists, and many others will help you along your journey. Reading this book is an enormous commitment to your health. Celebrate this huge step forward in your understanding!

You will do it! You will build confidence and success with strategies in this book and by working with your healthcare team.

The next chapter shows ways we can eat challenging solids with new confidence.

CHAPTER 11

HOW TO HANDLE DIFFICULT SOLIDS

When I met Hal, I wasn't quite prepared to hear my own 3-step method coming from a patient I'd never met. Hal had been dealing with trouble swallowing on and off for more than forty years. And he'd been tinkering with what helped (or didn't) for all that time. His gastroenterologist had done "all the scopes and balloons," and they would help, for months, or even years.

But what really helped, Hal explained, was what he called whetting his whistle. He always drinks something before he tries to eat any solid food. Then he starts out with foods that he knows won't cause him trouble, well before he moves on to meat, or bread, which he knew to be wary of. Most important of all, he said, was to follow each bite of solid food with a swallow of water. A retired plumber, Hal used a toilet flushing analogy to explain this process.

I was a little stunned to have my advice, derived from long personal experience, a medical degree, and a steady stream of patients with swallowing problems, come at me this way. Sometimes my 3-step process embarrasses me. After all, it is common sense and elementary—many patients could figure it out on their own. My hope, though, is to make the process more efficient, so no one has to spend four decades working this out for themselves.

Hal gave us a gift. People who struggle with esophagus attacks for ten or more years know one of my rules without me even asking. Most tell me Rule #2 first (easy solids before difficult solids). Some patients who've struggled for a couple of decades can tell me two rules. Hal, the plumber, struggled more than forty years to learn these three rules. When I met Hal, I knew I needed to share this. Reading this book can save you years of frustration.

As soon as Hal the plumber nailed down my third rule, I needed to ask him about a hundred more questions. Hal tinkered with his esophagus like he tinkers with plumbing and home-brewing beer. He experimented with different strategies and navigated this disease for almost a half-century. I listened to Hal's advice so I could share it with you.

Meeting thousands of patients struggling with food getting stuck, I learned to ask everyone what helps them. I keep mental notes and try out new ideas.

Hal confirmed many strategies and added more. I'll describe what I learned from Hal and other patients. This chapter contains patient suggestions and results of eighteen years of self-testing. These strategies help me eat meats and difficult solids, so you can, too.

There are two main take-home messages from this chapter. The first is to eat food you know won't cause problems.

The second take-home message is: do what works for you. You are an experimental laboratory. Be curious. Cut food into safe pieces you know you can swallow. This chapter presents many details, and my suggestions give you strategies, a general direction, and guardrails but not a specific destination. I empower you to take charge and find out what works best for you.

We introduced the Ogilvie scale for swallowing food in chapter 2. This scale offers suggestions about when to see your physician. If you're advancing on this scale, you need to let your physician know about these changes.

OGILVIE SCORE	LEVEL OF DIFFICULTY	SEE A DOCTOR?	HOW SOON TO SEE A PHYSICIAN?
0	No problems at all.	No.	Not applicable.
1	Avoid certain foods.	Yes.	This month.
2	Semi-solid diet only.	Yes.	This week.
3	Fluids only.	Yes.	Today or next business day. Consider urgent care if available.
4	No fluids pass at all.	Yes.	Visit ER now.

For example, if last month, you were avoiding meats and bread (Ogilvie 1), and this month, easy solids get stuck (Ogilvie 2); that's a change. Tell your doctor.

Eat food you know won't cause problems.

If you have undergone endoscopy or an esophagram and know that size, that's helpful. If your doctor passed 13 mm and 14 mm balloons, but the 15 mm balloon got stuck, that's important. Fourteen mm, a little bigger than 1/2 inch, should be safe for you. If the 12.7 mm barium tablet got stuck, then pieces of food larger than 12.7 mm will probably cause a problem. That's about half an inch in size. If the 10 mm scope wouldn't pass, then anything bigger than 10 mm will get stuck.

Follow your body's cues and be safe if you've never had these tests or you don't know for sure. Should something get stuck or feels like it almost gets stuck, you need to respect your body's signals.

RIGHT SIZE

You have two ways to get your food to the right size. One way is to cut it up outside your body. A second way is chew it up.

CUT IT UP

Cutting food to a safe size outside your body is safer. You have two main approaches. The first is obvious—cut your food on your plate. Humans have cut food to edible sizes for thousands of years. Another strategy is to cut food smaller before it hits your plate. A chef's knife and a cutting board is a superior cutting tool compared with a steak knife and a plate. Hal told me he's a stickler for sharp knives in his kitchen; good advice. Another excellent cutting tool is an onion holder, designed to stab an onion and hold it safely in place as you slice it into defined thickness slices. It is a multi-pronged device you can buy at most kitchen supply stores and Amazon. You can use it to cut meat like steak, chicken, or pork into thin slices. I cut my daughters' steak with it before they're ready for a steak knife.

CHEW, CHEW, CHEW

Chewing food to a safe size to swallow is the other big strategy after cutting it to a safe size. The benefit is you don't have to rely on a steak knife. You don't have to rely on a cutting board or a chef's knife. You always have your teeth. Think about camping trips. You don't bring your best knives. You might not have a plate. If you're at a cocktail party, you may not cut something into a safe bite.

You rely on your teeth. What if you don't have functioning teeth? Patients without teeth are at a significant disadvantage. You may struggle to chew solid bites into safe sizes.

Some pieces of food are too tough to chew into smaller pieces. You may be unsure if a bit is a safe size while you are chewing. Because of these disadvantages, try to cut up your food to a safe size before you eat. Be open to politely spitting out a piece of food you can't chew to a safe size. Spitting out a fatty chunk of steak beats an ER visit.

EAT MINDFULLY

Surgeons are a different breed. They do everything early and fast. As a medical student on general surgery at a VA hospital, I arrived around half past five in the morning to see patients and discuss them with the surgery team. Then the group of medical students, residents, and fellows eat breakfast at the hospital cafeteria. Surgeons do everything fast. Breakfast is no different. Shovel food down, and don't get left behind. I didn't chew a sausage link enough, and it got caught. I was speechless and looked down at my plate while my shoulders and back sagged. I stopped eating and grimaced. I tried swallowing milk. Rolling waves of pain. I wanted to walk away but knew the team was about to leave. I tried water. I waited as the waves of pain rolled through my chest. Five minutes later, the sausage passed. I skipped the rest of my breakfast, caught up with the team, and headed to the OR. Everything went by so fast I didn't process how embarrassed and ashamed I was. I struggled to swallow food surrounded by doctors and friends, and I still didn't reach out for help. I was still learning what was triggering my problem, so I shoved it back into my emotional basement and returned to being a medical student.

I was not eating mindfully and ignoring two problems. My esophagus and my emotional ignorance.

I shoveled food down as fast as I could. Fast eating doesn't go well if food gets stuck for you. You don't have to be the slowest eater at the table. The 3-step process of eating becomes a habit.

Slowing down eating allows your stomach to signal your brain you are full. You will overeat if you shovel food down and don't let your stomach signal your brain you're full.

DON'T OVERCOOK MEATS

You need to cook meat to a safe temperature. You probably prefer a specific internal temperature. A well-done steak challenges me to cut it up and swallow it in safe sizes. A medium-rare steak is easier to cut with a knife and chew with my teeth. I cook beef steaks to an internal temperature of medium-rare, 135 degrees F—you need a meat thermometer. These are inexpensive ($7-$15 basic, $20-$50 deluxe) devices to measure internal temperature. It removes the need to cut into meat to assess doneness—and tempt an esophagus attack like in chapter 7. A meat thermometer is a small cost compared with losing several overcooked steaks. It's nothing compared to your emergency room co-pay. Again, cook meat to a temperature where you are comfortable. The USDA offers food safety guidelines, and the science behind these guidelines is beyond this book.

WOOD PLANKS

We love wood planks and have used them for years. Many love the rind of flavor that develops around a steak to lock in juice called the char. Sometimes, char makes a steak harder to cut or chew. We avoid char and cook on wood planks. The steak doesn't contact hot grill grates, cooks the steak indirectly, and imparts a smoky flavor. If you want to sear, you can briefly sear the steak a minute or two on the grill, then switch to the wood planks. Grilling on water-soaked wood planks keeps steaks juicy.

SOFTER CUTS OF MEAT

Soft cuts of meat historically are more expensive. Filet mignon is the most delicate and costliest. We look for under-the-radar tender cuts of beef. The flat iron is popular. Butchers cut a flat iron steak from the cow's shoulder and represent the infraspinatus muscle. It goes by the nicknames of the "Butler's Cut" in the UK and Top Blade roast. The flat iron combines excellent flavor and tenderness. Another under-the-radar cut is the Teres Major. Butchers cut it from the shoulder and it goes by "Mock Tender," "Shoulder Tender," and "Petit Filet." After the filet mignon, it is the second-most tender cut of beef. It's half the cost of the filet mignon. The hanging tender steak is another under-the-radar cut. The "Butcher's Steak" earned its name because butchers kept it for themselves. Softer beef cuts allow you to enjoy beef with esophagus problems.

Another strategy is grass-fed cattle. In Iowa, local ranchers bring meat to Saturday farmer's markets. Your local meat locker supplies grass-fed meat. Try alternate sources of red meat—we love prairie-raised buffalo. We buy buffalo from a family in Rapid City, South Dakota, that raises them on the prairie. It is lower in fat than beef but remains tender and juicy when grilled. Consider cooking buffalo on wood planks with a temperature gauge to avoid char.

FISH

Fish is a terrific protein. Our favorite is Alaskan rockfish. We buy seafood from a family in Ninilchik, Alaska, that sells outstanding fish and seafood. Rockfish grills well and keeps moisture. It is flaky at a more reasonable price. When fish cuts with a fork, it will be easy to chew. Monterey Bay Aquarium Seafood Watch ranks Alaskan Rockfish as a "Best Choice" for sustainability, their highest award. We grill rockfish on wood planks with a temperature gauge. Rockfish is 3/4-1.5 inch thick, so it's easy to use a temperature probe.

My general principle with fish and seafood is to find sustainable fork-tender options. We love scallops in our home and avoid overcooking. Charleston, South Carolina, was our home for five years, and we struggle to find shrimp as good as the Lowcountry. I love shrimp as a sustainable protein. Thousands of seafood choices inspire intriguing meals. You'll find healthy options your esophagus will love!

COOKING METHODS

If you search for "Acid Reflux Cookbook" on Amazon, you'll find 409 different results. Vast resources help you bravely eat yummy food. Here are some general principles for cooking success.

Cooking any meat a long time at low heat results in fork-tender proteins. Dutch oven, Crock Pot, Instant Pot, sous vide, and Traeger's grills are options. Don't feel restricted to cookbooks designed for your particular diagnosis (Acid Reflux, Barrett's Esophagus, Gastric Sleeve, etc.). With a goal of fork-tender protein, you can get there from many routes.

We're mindful to know where we get our proteins. In central Iowa, we can buy locally raised meat and poultry. In large cities, search out butcher shops and describe you're looking for tender, humanely raised, grass-fed beef, pork, chicken, etc. If all else fails, you can search out families in America that raise animals and ship frozen meat, poultry, or fish to your door.

Embrace eating the protein you want, whatever it is. Beef, pork, chicken, buffalo, and fish are all options.

Envision how it will feel to eat the meat you would like and cut it with a fork. You'll eat more confidently and successfully! You'll build success, knowing your goal is tender meat.

NON-ANIMAL OPTIONS

Protein is a necessary macro-nutrient. You can eat enough protein from non-meat or plant-based sources. Even if you love meat, find ways to add protein to your diet with non-meat options. Beans, legumes, chickpeas, and edamame are all great non-meat proteins. As a bonus, they're small and rarely trigger esophagus attacks.

Tofu is another sustainable protein. Tofu replaces or complements meats as a sustainable protein. Consider tofu for anyone who struggles to swallow difficult solids. Consistencies vary from soft to super-firm. We prefer super-firm because the texture is closer to firm fish or meat. If you struggle with firm solids, more delicate silken tofu is like a block of soft cheese. Cut tofu to the right size for your esophagus. If your esophagus is narrow, dice your tofu into 5 mm cubes. Food processors are great for this. Tofu may inspire you to add more protein back in your diet because you can always chop it smaller.

The Impossible Burger and Beyond Meat are meat-like proteins made from plants. Sounds good, right? Plants are sustainable, right? Good for our planet? Maybe not good for us. In chapter 12, we'll dive into eosinophilic esophagitis and the unknowns about processed foods. For now, file away the idea that highly processed foods might not be the best choice for folks with esophagus problems.

PROTEIN SUPPLEMENTS

A few patients reach the point they can no longer eat solid food. Perhaps it is severe esophageal stenosis refractory to dilation (more on that in chapter 12). Some have esophageal cancer and cannot eat solid food. We still need protein in our diet, and protein powders or protein shakes help. For some with mild esophageal narrowing, protein supplements can be a tasty way to increase protein intake.

Protein shakes occasionally challenge me. Milk blended with frozen bananas thickens to the consistency of ice cream and gets stuck. Since I prepare protein shakes in a blender, nothing is big enough to get stuck for long. Another option is swallowing something hot to thaw the shake, and it will pass.

You must see your physician if you're struggling and can only drink protein shakes. Ensure shakes are the most available meal replacement shake. Lean on your physician or a dietician for more options.

Dairy-based options like yogurt are a final protein supplement that also adds calcium to your diet. But, dairy products are a potential cause of eosinophilic esophagitis. We'll dive into this in chapter 12. Many non-dairy yogurt-like protein options exist than ever before.

BLENDERIZE FOOD

If you have progressed so far along the Ogilvie scale that you can only eat semi-solid or liquid-based food, you must see a physician. Options still exist. One of my daughters has a severe heart problem, and we have fed her through a tube since she was four months old. We went through a phase where we blended natural foods in a powerful blender and injected it into her stomach. It opened my eyes to both opportunities and struggles families endure.

Infants as young as a year old can receive blenderized diets, but only guided by a registered dietician or nutritionist. Feel reassured you can meet nutritional needs in a variety of ways. Physicians, speech therapists, and dieticians work to help people eat on their own.

TIME TESTED STRATEGIES

Remember Hal the plumber earlier in this chapter? Hal harnessed curiosity about plumbing and experimented until he solved his swallowing problem. Hal already knew he needed to figure out what works for him. You're reading Hal's strategies and other patients' solutions that I've tested.

There are thousands of solutions to the various problems your esophagus can cause you. Adopt Hal's experimental attitude. Grant yourself curiosity and space to try some of these solutions. Lean into your issue. Face it and own it. Be inspired by your ability to triumph over difficult solids. Now move on to chapter 12 and learn about specific esophagus diagnoses and how these strategies apply.

CHAPTER 12

DIAGNOSES ASSOCIATED WITH ESOPHAGUS ATTACKS

After Easter, the other big holiday our whole family gets together for is Thanksgiving. So much has changed for me between those two days this year! When I finally saw the doctor, it was such a relief just to know I was getting help. Even with all the tests I had to go through, and the pills I take, and the changes I needed to make, the whole process was so worth it. Anything in life that's worthwhile takes work. Raising this whole family wasn't always easy, but I wouldn't trade it for anything. Losing my son is still the worst pain I've ever had, but working through my grief brought some positive things. Compared to things like that, facing my fear that it could be cancer, and fixing my swallowing, was pretty easy, I guess. And now I have good knowledge of how my body works, a diagnosis I understand, an eating system that works, and a GI doctor I trust to help me out when I need it. I'm finally talking with the people important to me about my experience, and that makes it so much easier to live with! And with those answers and that support, I'm free of the anxiety, uncertainty, and embarrassment caused by problems swallowing. It's been a challenge, for sure, and I give myself credit for getting a handle on all this. That's why my answer to our Thanksgiving "what-are-you-grateful-for" go-round was, "Eating!"

Michelle, who we met in an earlier chapter, was thriving with the new knowledge and strategies she'd learned by finally seeking medical treatment for her esophagus problems. For many people, their solutions lie in the topics covered in all the other chapters in this book. For some people, though, their journey takes them more deeply into the medical world, so, for those who will find it helpful, this chapter maps out the territory. We'll cover all the conditions I know my 3 steps method (Liquid Before Solid, Easy Solids Before Difficult Solids, Flush with Liquid) helps.

We're re-entering the medical world. Be ready to learn about conditions, treatments, and surgeries. I'll explain how the 3-step process from earlier chapters applies to each diagnosis.

You'll learn new medical terms.

For each, I'll explain the problem. Since cancer is on everyone's mind, you'll learn what's cancer or a precursor to cancer. You'll know whether the 3-step process helps. You'll learn if a proton pump inhibitor is part of the initial treatment and if it's necessary long-term. You'll learn if surgery plays a role in treatment.

One saying from medical school: repetition is the key to learning. You will gain knowledge and confidence as you cement your understanding. In this chapter, you'll read about simple and common problems before you learn about rare disorders.

This chapter isn't required reading. Tackle as much as you wish. Sections of this chapter are diagnoses I hope you never hear (esophageal cancer, Barrett's esophagus, etc.). Consider this chapter an encyclopedia of esophagus problems. Don't get hung up on understanding everything 100 percent. My goal remains to make medical content accessible to everyone. Don't let medical terms intimidate you. We're in this together. I'm your guide and you've made it this far with me.

DIAGNOSIS: REFLUX (AKA GASTROESOPHAGEAL REFLUX OR GER)

Reflux is gastric contents moving upward into the esophagus, throat, or even your mouth. Most patients don't notice reflux until it's in their mouth and causes a foul taste. Others sense reflux in their esophagus or throat.

It's not cancer!

Painless reflux occurs in adults. It happens to me, and I don't worry.

We consider reflux with pain, discomfort, or other negative symptoms to be gastroesophageal reflux disease (i.e., GERD).

If you only have reflux without other problems, consider my 3 steps informational.

Lifestyle changes prevent uncomplicated reflux from progressing to a disease (GERD).

A proton pump inhibitor (PPI) isn't necessary to treat uncomplicated occasional reflux.

Surgery won't help uncomplicated reflux and isn't necessary.

DIAGNOSIS: GERD (GASTROESOPHAGEAL REFLUX DISEASE)

GERD is gastric contents moving upward into the esophagus, throat, or even mouth with pain, discomfort, or another negative symptom. Doctors can diagnose GERD when problems attributed to GERD develop, like chronic throat clearing, hoarseness, asthma, aspiration pneumonia, chronic ear infections, chronic sinus disease and postnasal drip. Michelle's

Easter ham caused an esophagus attack back in chapter 7, but now she's in control of her GERD with better understanding, treatment, and help from her physician.

This isn't cancer.

Treat GERD with lifestyle modification and proton pump inhibitors (PPI) to heal the esophagus and prevent progression.

If you have GERD and no esophagus attacks, consider my 3 steps informational. Don't worry about the 3 steps unless food gets stuck.

Treat your GERD, and you shouldn't progress to a stricture. Most people use PPIs for a month or two months and stop. If the pain doesn't return, your doctor assumes your esophagus healed. Ongoing PPI therapy isn't necessary unless painful reflux (i.e., GERD) returns, or your doctor recommends staying on it for another reason.

Surgery is only helpful for GERD in severe cases.

What really causes GERD? Since 1935, no one questioned stomach acid as the villain. In the last five years, new data suggested your immune system is the villain.

Immune system? Causing GERD? What?

Confused?

I was.

I'll explain.

We thought stomach acid injured or killed surface esophagus cells. More acid killed layer after layer of cells. Doctors thought as layers died, the deepest layer of cells created different acid-resistant cells. Like our skin creates callouses at sites of overuse, doctors thought your esophagus made different cells resistant to acid injury.

Researchers in Texas tested this idea from 2013 to 2015. They found patients with documented esophagitis. All patients took a PPI twice daily. The researchers checked the esophagus and took pieces of tissue to prove the PPI-treated esophagus was normal before the experiment.

Then, the researchers took away the patient's PPI for two weeks.

All patients underwent repeat biopsy at nine and sixteen days.

Then all patients went back on their PPI.

What did they find? Every patient re-injured their esophagus. At biopsy, they found clear evidence of reflux. They also found the patient's immune system attacked the esophagus. All patients also reported their reflux symptoms returned.

The researchers presume the esophagus cells sent out cytokines. Cytokines are our body's signal for help—like a sinking ship sending an SOS signal or a 911 call in the modern era. Cytokines attract immune cells. They found immune cell damage was much worse than acid damage.

Does this matter? Not really. We don't know if acid is the bad actor or an overzealous immune response is the real villain, but stomach acid hitting your esophagus is the root cause. You must stop the reflux. PPIs treat the problem either way. Remember, these patients were successfully treated with PPIs. If your immune system is the villain, drug companies will develop new medicines to block or blunt the immune response. Some GERD patients now receive immunotherapy designed for cancer patients to test this idea.

But I go back to the original idea.

Stop. Reflux.

If you can do that, you can skip the pills. That's why chapter 9 comes before chapter 10. Lifestyle changes trump pills.

GERD tying to the immune system intensely interests me because it links EoE and GERD. In EoE, eosinophils infiltrate the esophagus. Eosinophils are immune cells. In this trial, lymphocytes infiltrate the esophagus. Lymphocytes are immune cells. See the link? In both EoE and GERD, immune cells infiltrate our esophagus, reduce esophagus function, and cause esophagus attacks.

Now, why eosinophils in younger patients and lymphocytes in older patients? We don't know. We're struggling with puzzle pieces that don't neatly fit together. More about EoE later in this chapter.

DIAGNOSIS: HIATAL HERNIA

Part of the stomach leaves the abdominal cavity and enters the chest cavity. The muscular junction between the esophagus and stomach doesn't stay closed, and gastroesophageal reflux happens more.

A hiatal hernia is a structural problem—not cancer. I reassured Michelle that her hiatal hernia wasn't cancer or pre-cancerous. I could see her shoulders drop and calm come over her when I told her.

Doctors aren't sure why a hiatal hernia develops. Our best guess is over-eating stretches the stomach at the diaphragm, injures small ligaments, and allows the stomach to slip upward into the chest cavity. So, try to avoid over-eating.

The 3-step process helps patients with hiatal hernias.

Doctors use PPIs to treat hiatal-hernia associated GERD. If you have a hiatal hernia but have no pain or problems, you don't have GERD and shouldn't need a PPI. There's no role for a PPI for an uncomplicated hiatal hernia.

Surgery has a limited role for a hiatal hernia. Surgeons consider fixing a hiatal hernia if you do everything in your power to change your lifestyle and maximize pill-based therapy and still suffer GERD. Failing medical therapy and a massive volume of reflux are also reasons to consider surgery. Severe esophagitis, a benign stricture, or Barrett's esophagus are other reasons to consider surgery.

Most surgeons do a Nissen fundoplication to fix a hiatal hernia. That's a mouthful. I explain this surgery later in this chapter.

DIAGNOSIS: GASTRIC VOLVULUS

A hiatal hernia develops and increases in size. The hernia enlarges, and ligaments holding the stomach in place fail. The stomach migrates upward into the chest cavity and flips vertically or horizontally. Gastric volvulus can cause obstruction requiring urgent or emergency surgery.

Gastric volvulus has an ominous name, but it's not cancer.

You must consider surgery if gastric volvulus stops you from eating. See a surgeon if you have gastric volvulus and trouble with food getting stuck. My 3-step process may help, but you need to know how obstructed your stomach is.

A PPI may help with esophagitis but will not fix the volvulus. There's a minor role for long-term PPI treatment for a gastric volvulus without GERD. If you have chronic GERD with gastric volvulus, there may be a role for long-term PPI use.

DIAGNOSIS: CRICOPHARYNGEUS MUSCLE HYPERTROPHY (AKA PROMINENT CRICOPHARYNGEUS MUSCLE OR CRICOPHARYNGEUS ACHALASIA)

The cricopharyngeus muscle forms part of the upper esophageal sphincter. This muscle contracts and holds the upper esophagus closed. Relaxing the cricopharyngeus muscle opens the upper esophageal sphincter. Recent research suggests GERD worsens cricopharyngeus muscle hypertrophy. GERD may make the cricopharyngeus work harder and get thicker. A thick cricopharyngeus muscle may contribute to problems swallowing and cause the sense that food gets stuck in the upper esophagus.

Physicians believe a Zenker diverticulum develops from cricopharyngeus muscle hypertrophy. Imagine you reflux up your esophagus and the cricopharyngeus muscle does its job and stops reflux from entering your throat or trachea.

The acid and partially digested food has to go somewhere. The weakest place in the neighborhood is a thin layer of tissue. Over time, with repeated episodes, a small outpouching develops. If this happens over and over, the diverticulum gets bigger. It can become so large food gets stuck inside the diverticulum.

This is not cancer. If you have cricopharyngeus muscle hypertrophy or a Zenker diverticulum, see a gastroenterologist. They will assess whether you need treatment, and which treatment is optimal.

Your GI doctor may inject Botox in the muscle to relax it, but this may increase reflux. Your doctor may dilate the muscle with a balloon, but this too may increase reflux.

The 3-step process of eating should help.

Patients with this likely have GERD, so expect questions regarding GERD symptoms. A GI doctor performs endoscopy to evaluate this condition. If GERD is present, PPI therapy is necessary. You need long-term PPI therapy if GERD persists. If GERD resolves, no need for long-term PPI therapy.

Surgical approaches exist. A surgeon can do a myotomy to cut the muscle. A myotomy is a more invasive treatment reserved if endoscopic Botox injections or balloon dilations fail. Most patients start with Botox or balloon dilation before a considering a myotomy. A surgeon can remove a Zenker diverticulum if it is large or causes other problems.

DIAGNOSIS: ESOPHAGEAL STRICTURE

An esophageal stricture narrows the esophagus, causing food to get stuck and pain after swallowing. GERD is the most common cause, but eosinophilic esophagitis or other diseases of the esophagus can cause a stricture. Esophagus strictures are more commonly benign than cancer—a biopsy is necessary to differentiate. For the rest of our discussion on esophagus strictures, assume the stricture is non-cancerous (aka benign).

A stricture may be simple or complex, and benign, refractory, or recurrent. A simple stricture occurs in the distal esophagus and is smooth, short, and straight. A 10 mm endoscope passes through it.

A complex stricture is long, narrow, tortuous, or part of a large hiatal hernia. Patients with a stricture need an esophagus dilation, so please see a GI doctor if you have a stricture. During dilation, a balloon-like device called a bougie passes through the esophagus and dilates it. Other doctors use an inflatable medical balloon to dilate the esophagus. More complex strictures require careful attention during dilation.

Esophagus dilation helps the patient swallow food normally again. Most doctors follow the rule of 3's of dilation. They dilate only 3 mm per session. Let's say your esophagus is 12 mm. They will pass a 12 mm bougie without a problem. Then they pass 13 mm, 14 mm, and 15 mm bougies against mild resistance. They stop dilating. Many doctors agree 16 mm or bigger is the dilation goal. A patient who dilated to 15 mm will return in a week or 2 for another dilation. Michelle needed two dilation sessions to improve her stricture and swallowing.

GI doctors biopsy the esophagus before or after dilation, if they believe biopsy is safe. Biopsy means to take a tiny piece of tissue for microscopic analysis. Biopsy ensures no other process like eosinophilic esophagitis or Barrett's esophagus is present.

Patients who undergo a dilation usually have PPI therapy with omeprazole 20 mg twice daily for one year to reduce the need for later dilations and control reflux. This book originated to help patients with esophageal strictures, so the 3-step approach to eating helps.

Surgery does not help most patients. Esophageal cancer is one exception—surgery is usually part of their therapy plan. If dilation doesn't fix the stricture, surgery may be a consideration.

DIAGNOSIS: RECURRENT ESOPHAGEAL STRICTURE

A recurrent stricture dilates to 14 mm or larger but in less than four weeks cannot keep that diameter and needs re-dilation. In other words, the esophagus narrowing opens but narrows back down in four weeks.

This is not cancer.

If you have a recurrent stricture, you're seeing a gastroenterologist. Keep at it. They will re-dilate you several times, but they may discuss other options. The most important question to ask is whether they see inflammation in your esophagus. If you still have esophagus inflammation, they must maximize PPI therapy and lifestyle changes. If you have no inflammation during dilation, they may inject steroid medicines at the stricture. Steroids are potent medicines to suppress inflammation, fibrosis, and stricture recurrence. If steroids don't work, an endoscopic incision is usually the next choice. We cover endoscopic incision later in this chapter.

The 3-step process for eating is vital. These patients need every advantage to improve swallowing.

PPIs are important. If you have a stricture, take PPIs when diagnosed and plan to take them long-term, directed by your gastroenterologist.

Surgery is a last choice for a stricture. Physicians suspect inflammation contributes to recurrent strictures. Surgery causes abundant inflammation and injury to the esophagus. It may make everything worse.

DIAGNOSIS: REFRACTORY ESOPHAGEAL STRICTURE

A refractory stricture will not dilate past 14 mm in five dilation sessions in two weeks. In other words, no matter how hard we try, we cannot dilate the esophagus to 14 mm in two weeks.

It's not cancer.

Keep seeing your gastroenterologist. They will re-dilate you, but they will discuss other options if dilation fails. Similar to the recurrent stricture, esophagus inflammation cannot be present. Inflammation signals your doctor to maximize your PPI dosing. Inflammation tells us you need to keep working to optimize lifestyle choices. They inject steroids into a recurrent stricture if no inflammation is present. If steroids don't work, an endoscopic incision is next.

The 3-step process for eating is critical. PPI is a cornerstone for initial and long-term therapy of a refractory stricture.

Surgery is still a last-ditch choice.

PROCEDURE/SURGERY: ENDOSCOPIC ESOPHAGUS INCISION

If a stricture doesn't respond to balloons and steroids, the gastroenterologist can cut the esophagus on the inside to open it.

This is a cutting procedure, not cancer.

An endoscopic incision is a newer procedure, and I would tell family members to find a physician who performs and teaches this procedure. Consider endoscopic incision only after failure of dilation with a balloon or a balloon-like device. One article specified three dilation sessions with a balloon or balloon-like device, and three sessions with a steroid injection before contemplating endoscopic incision. If a stricture persists after six sessions, then consider endoscopic incision.

The 3-step process of eating helps patients with a severe stricture.

A PPI is a cornerstone of therapy for patients who need an endoscopic incision. If endoscopic incision and esophageal stent placement fail, surgery is a choice.

My wife and I understand advanced therapies like endoscopic incision should occur with experienced doctors, usually at large hospitals.

Here's our brief story. My four-month-old son died of an extremely rare disease called pulmonary vein stenosis (PVS) at a children's hospital in Nebraska. The physicians and nurses did everything they could, but Ben was too sick. Ben looked well aside from struggles to gain weight when doctors admitted him to the hospital. Ben died that week. I'd never felt emotional pain like that. Doctors in Iowa later diagnosed our rainbow daughter Caroline with PVS when she was three months old. My wife and I were desperate to give Caroline any chance we could. When offered two hospitals for Caroline, we chose the biggest, University of Iowa. We thought her future was bleak. The University of Iowa doctors didn't offer treatment. But they offered to transfer Caroline to Boston Children's Hospital for a new treatment program for PVS. One miracle followed another, and Caroline is almost five years old while I write this. She illustrates the most experienced physicians best treat rare diseases. For routine problems, your local hospital is nearly always the best choice.

DEVICE/DIAGNOSIS: ESOPHAGUS STENT

A stent is a plastic or metal device to open a narrow part of the esophagus.

A stent is a medical device, not a diagnosis.

GI doctors place stents for patients with esophageal cancer

when needed. A few patients with benign strictures get removable or biodegradable stents. If your gastroenterologist considers a stent, your disease hasn't responded to standard treatments. I'm sure both you and your doctor share disappointment if your stricture fails usual therapy. There are bare-metal stents that look like a metal scaffold. Avoid these. They work for a few patients, but the complication rate is high. The esophagus grows into bare-metal stents and narrows again. Plastic stents covered by a membrane prevent the esophagus from growing into the stent and re-narrowing. These are better than bare-metal stents.

Two trials with 202 patients tested plastic stents. Fifty percent of the patients receiving these stents did not need re-dilation. Plastic-covered stents hold promise because these patients failed conservative treatments.

Migration is the biggest problem with covered stents. They move into the stomach, cause an obstruction, and need urgent or emergent removal. Twenty-four percent and 31 percent of these stents migrated in two studies, so almost one in three patients needed urgent stent removal. One patient died from major bleeding associated with a stent.

The newest option is a biodegradable stent. These stents naturally break down in three to four months. Patients usually do well for three months, then have a stenosis recurrence. When the stent decays, you get another stent. Major complications occurred in 29 percent after one stent, 8 percent after two stents and 28 percent after three stents. There's no perfect stent; follow your doctor's advice on stents. Consider going to an experienced GI doctor if you need a stent.

The 3-step process of eating is important for patients who need a stent in their esophagus. Patients with esophagus stents need PPIs after stent placement and long-term.

Surgery represents the final option if stents fail—or surgery isn't an option.

DIAGNOSIS: EOSINOPHILIC ESOPHAGITIS (EOE)

When Riley realized the pain after swallowing that bite of chicken was enough to make her hunch over the table, clutching her chest, she started running through possible solutions in her mind. She could try milk, but that was sure to make it feel worse, despite what she'd been told about sipping liquids. Was she going to have to go throw up, just to get the food unstuck?

This can't be normal, she told herself. I need to go back to the doctor. Getting angry about it isn't helping me any, and I need to figure this out. Could I have an infection? An allergy? I could just not eat meat until I understand why I get such pain when I swallow, but I need a better solution than just 'no chicken.'

Riley was at the beginning of her diagnostic journey, but

eventually she would learn she has eosinophilic esophagitis or EoE. As diseases go, eosinophilic esophagitis is new. First described in 1993, doctors find EoE in 12-15 percent of adults with dysphasia. If food gets stuck for you, one in six has EoE. Under 40? Your chances of EoE rise. Allergies challenge you? Your EoE chances rise more.

Eosinophils are immune cells that fight disease and cause EoE. The eosinophils migrate into the esophagus wall, cause narrowing, and diminish esophagus contraction. GI doctors biopsy the esophagus, so they remove many cells in a biopsy. Pathologists, doctors who specialize in looking at tiny pieces of tissue under a microscope, count how many eosinophils they see in one view. If they see over fifteen, that's the definition of EoE.

As you learned in the GERD section earlier in this chapter, researchers are starting to believe our immune system may contribute to GERD. Lymphocytes, an immune cell that fights disease, are found in the esophagus in higher numbers than expected after only two weeks of active GERD. Lymphocytes in GERD and eosinophils in EoE? Is there a link between our immune system and these esophagus diseases? Probably.

EoE is not cancer and not pre-cancerous.

Doctors recognize EoE commonly causes food to get stuck.

About 250,000 in the USA have EoE. We discover EoE at esophagus biopsy more often today than twenty years ago, and physicians don't know why.

Experts think a global change in our diet triggered EoE. Our available data on EoE points to our food supply. Genetically modified foods? Pesticides? Fewer bacteria, mold, or fungi in our diets? Chemicals/steroids in our milk? Something else? No one knows.

The esophagus may look healthy when EoE is present, so it's a tricky diagnosis. Sometimes, the only hint EoE lurks in a patient's esophagus is a stricture. However, a study from the Mayo Clinic showed gastroenterologists miss 75 percent of the strictures less than 13 mm in size, so even a stricture may be hard to see. New guidelines suggest the GI doctor takes four to six biopsies, even if the esophagus looks normal. Biopsy a normal esophagus? After an esophagus attack from food getting stuck—it's critical!

If you have EoE, you may see a gastroenterologist, an allergist, and a dietician. All three help treat EoE.

A PPI is a first-line therapy for EoE. If the eosinophils in the esophagus during biopsy go down or resolve, the GI doctor reduces or eliminates the PPI. If the PPI doesn't help, your GI doctor will recommend eliminating foods from your diet. Swallowing a steroid medicine mixed with a thickening agent like honey also treats EoE. Researchers test other EoE drug treatments now.

We used to eliminate six foods to stop EoE. Removing cow's milk, wheat, egg, soy, peanut/tree nuts, and fish/shellfish cured many. There are two problems. One, that's a super restrictive diet! Two, it means forty-two weeks of diet modifications, until you KNOW what triggers your EoE. It starts with six weeks of total elimination, then reintroduces six foods, one-by-one, once every six weeks, with scopes after each introduction. (Six to seven scopes in total.)

We knew nuts and fish were rarely a problem, so doctors eventually settled on a four-food elimination diet for adults. Here's how it works.

You start with a scope that shows EoE with more than fifteen eosinophils per high powered field, a technical term for pathologists. Just remember, fifteen is too many.

Next, eliminate four foods from your diet. People knock out dairy products, wheat, egg, and legumes/soy from their diet for six weeks.

Not just milk. Anything that uses milk as an ingredient. Anything that uses wheat or flour as an ingredient. Same goes for eggs and soy/legumes. It is restrictive. But we need to figure out what's causing EoE.

Then, re-scope and prove eosinophils went away (or less than fifteen).

Then, you reintroduce foods one-by-one. Wheat returns first. Re-introduce wheat products into your diet for six weeks. Then, re-scope and biopsy. If no EoE, dairy products were brought back. If EoE returned (eosinophils more than fifteen) when a food was reintroduced, it was labeled an "EoE trigger" and permanently eliminated from the patient's diet.

There's confusion about EoE triggers. When chicken, beef, bread, or sushi cause an esophagus attack, they usually aren't an EoE trigger. That's a food that got stuck, caused pain, and you were miserable. Some people think the act of food getting stuck and causing an esophagus attack triggers their EoE. It's not. These are different things.

The foods that are EoE triggers (cow's milk, wheat, soy, eggs) pass through your esophagus fine. Something about this food causes eosinophils to bum-rush your esophagus and cause problems.

With this approach, 54 percent of patients achieved remission. In other words, EoE went away, and swallowing became normal again.

Milk was the most common trigger in 50 percent of patients.

Egg was a trigger for 36 percent, wheat triggered 31 percent, and legumes or soy triggered 18 percent.

If the four-food elimination diet wasn't successful, they moved to a six-food elimination diet and took away all nuts and fish/seafood. A few more patients responded to the six-food elimination diet.

If eliminating foods doesn't work, doctors move on to treating with steroids. For adults and children, physicians use steroids typically prescribed for asthma. Rather than inhale the steroid medicine, the patient swallows steroid down the esophagus. Budesonide mixed with Splenda creates a thick slurry the patient swallows.

Don't eat for thirty minutes after swallowing the steroid so it stays in contact with the esophagus longer.

Fluticasone is another steroid option. Ever seen the asthma inhalers that you push on the top and a puff of medicine is breathed in? Same thing, but the patient DOESN'T breathe in. They just puff it in their mouth and dry swallow the medicine. Same as the other medicine, avoid eating for thirty minutes so the medicine stays in the esophagus longer.

About half or 50 percent of patients heal their EoE after three months of steroid treatment. Keep in mind, the patients who go to steroid treatment failed or couldn't tolerate the food elimination diet, so they have some of the worst cases of EoE.

What about kids? The four-food elimination diet approach works for kids, too. A trial achieved remission for 64 percent of kids. Cow's milk triggered 85 percent, egg triggered 35 percent, wheat triggered 33 percent, and soy triggered 19 percent. Thirty-eight percent of patients had more than one trigger, so the percentages don't add up to 100 percent. They took the same approach as for adults.

If you have EoE and features of GERD, the PPI is used to treat the GERD. Your GI doctor may not dilate your esophagus until GERD resolves. Surgery is not part of EoE treatment.

This disease happens more commonly in adults than children, but EoE happens in kids. We don't know the cause for EoE in adults or kids yet. This book and my 3-step eating process help adults with EoE but isn't designed for pediatric patients.

DIAGNOSIS: ESOPHAGEAL MOTILITY DISORDER

This book primarily focuses on esophagus narrowing like a pinched garden hose. A motility disorder is different. Motility disorders are problems with how the esophagus muscles contract or problems with nerves sending messages to or from the esophagus. Ten to thirty uncommon diseases of the esophagus cause motility disorders. Maybe the esophagus muscles squeeze too hard? Perhaps they're too weak? Do the muscles squeeze at all? A variety of abnormal contraction patterns make swallowing difficult and cause food to get stuck.

This isn't cancer. If your doctor thinks you have a motility disorder, you need special tests.

Remember high-resolution manometry from chapter 3? This helps your doctor diagnose your motility problem. The motility diagnosis determines the best treatment. You will follow your gastroenterologist's lead. If your motility problem involves nerves, your GI doctor may refer you to a neurologist. These doctors help patients with nerve problems.

People with motility disorders swallow better using the 3-step process in this book.

There's no role for PPIs for most motility problems—unless you also have GERD.

Surgery does not help patients with motility disorders.

SURGERY: NISSEN FUNDOPLICATION

We're switching gears and heading into surgeries to fix esophagus problems. To fix a hiatal hernia, a surgeon moves the stomach from the chest cavity back into the abdomen cavity. Then they repair the hole in the diaphragm. Surgeons call this the Nissen fundoplication.

This is surgery, not cancer. Other operations to fix a hiatal hernia are variations of a Nissen.

Seek out an experienced surgeon. Listen to their discussion of challenges during recovery and surgical risks. Balance surgical risks and challenges during recovery against your current problems. Many patients benefit from this surgery, but a few trade one set of problems for other problems.

The 3-step process helps patients with hiatal hernias.

Follow your surgeon's advice on taking a PPI before surgery. After surgery, a PPI is unnecessary because a Nissen usually eliminates GERD.

SURGERY: GASTRIC BYPASS

A gastric bypass transports food past the stomach and proximal bowel to reduce caloric intake and decrease nutrient absorption for weight loss.

This isn't cancer.

Gastric bypass surgery has revolutionized weight loss for

extremely obese individuals. To consider this surgery, patients must:

1. have a body mass index (BMI) over 40;
2. weigh over 100 pounds above ideal body weight, or
3. have a BMI over thirty-five and an obesity-related diagnosis, including GERD, type II diabetes, hypertension, sleep apnea, osteoarthritis, high lipid levels, or non-alcoholic fatty liver disease. With a BMI over thirty-five and any of those diagnoses, most surgeons consider you a candidate for gastric bypass or another weight-loss surgery.

Surgeons have performed gastric bypass over a decade. Gastric bypass re-routes your food. You lose weight for two reasons. First, the surgeon creates a smaller stomach, the size of your fist. You feel full sooner, and you must eat small meals. Second, after food leaves your new stomach, it bypasses several feet of bowel through a new loop. Bypassing intestine reduces the calories absorbed. To learn more, talk to a surgeon.

You will eat smaller more frequent meals after gastric bypass. Your surgery team will give you a specific diet to meet your nutritional needs. You shouldn't have problems with food getting stuck in your esophagus after surgery. If you find food gets stuck, work with your surgeon and a gastroenterologist to figure out why. Is it a problem in the new stomach pouch? An issue with the loop of bowel brought up to the stomach pouch? Esophagus problem? Infrequent problems develop after a gastric bypass, but your surgeon will help uncover the cause.

Doctors rarely use PPIs after gastric bypass surgery.

SURGERY: SLEEVE GASTRECTOMY

This surgery reduces stomach size to decrease food intake and cause weight loss.

This isn't cancer—it's a surgery.

Sleeve gastrectomy is a popular weight-loss surgery. It is less complicated than a gastric bypass. A surgeon reduces stomach size, so you feel full sooner, and you eat less. Gastric bypass detours your food beyond several feet of gut whereas sleeve gastrectomy reduces stomach size.

It is uncommon for food to get stuck after sleeve gastrectomy. If this happens, follow up with your surgeon and a gastroenterologist to discover why.

The 3-step eating process may help.

Doctors don't use PPIs much after this surgery.

POP QUIZ

Q. The 3-step process of swallowing helps patients with these conditions EXCEPT:

1. Children with EoE.

2. Adults with EoE.

3. Adults with a mild esophageal stricture.

4. Adults with a small hiatal hernia and GERD.

Answer: 1. Children with EoE. The 3-step process of eating applies to adults but not children.

DIAGNOSIS: LYE OR ACID STRICTURE (AKA CHEMICAL STRICTURE)

Strong acid or strong base chemicals damage the esophagus forever. Battery acid (highly acidic, pH 1.0) or Draino or Clorox bleach (highly basic, pH 11) is ingested accidentally by children or adults for self-harm. The esophagus develops a stricture that limits eating.

Chemical strictures aren't cancer, but this injury increases cancer risk.

Never ingest a powerful acid or a strong base like Clorox. If you do or you're helping a friend, make sure they see a GI or ENT doctor. They help manage long-term problems stemming from this injury. They will need specialized care for the rest of their life because of the ingestion. Don't lose hope. Many treatments, including balloon-like dilation and medications, help chemical strictures.

The 3-step process should help as long as a gastroenterologist endorses it.

GI doctors strongly recommend a PPI after the injury to help heal the esophagus injury but not long-term.

Surgeons rarely remove the esophagus for a chemical stricture.

DIAGNOSIS: ACHALASIA

In achalasia, the distal esophagus sphincter contracts too forcefully and won't relax. This problem is considered a motility disorder. Achalasia makes food, pills, or even liquid obstruct. The esophagus above the too-tight sphincter dilates and doesn't squeeze well.

This isn't cancer.

See a GI doctor for achalasia. A variety of treatments may help. Isosorbide is a long-acting nitrate that may help relax the tight muscle. Nifedipine is a calcium channel blocker that may also help. Dilating the too-tight sphincter with a balloon-like device treats achalasia.

Surgical treatments like the Heller myotomy or the peroral

endoscopic myotomy (POEM) cut the sphincter muscle, so it opens better.

The 3-step process of eating helps with achalasia.

A PPI usually isn't part of basic achalasia treatment. Because the distal esophagus squeezes too forcefully, it prevents reflux. After achalasia dilation or surgery, most patients get a PPI.

DIAGNOSIS: BARRETT'S ESOPHAGUS

In Barrett's esophagus, the cells of the distal esophagus change into the cells that line the stomach. Doctors think chronic acid exposure from GERD causes the change.

Barrett's esophagus is a pre-malignant, or pre-cancerous, condition. If you have Barrett's esophagus, your risk of esophageal cancer is 0.1–0.5 percent per year. The risk is lower, 0.1–0.25 percent per year, if the changes in the cells are low grade. If doctors find high-grade cellular changes, your cancer risk rises closer to 0.5 percent per year. If nothing changes, Barrett's esophagus slowly changes to esophageal cancer.

Finding Barrett's esophagus has a silver lining. Doctors found your cancer early. Cancer discovered early is easier to treat.

See your gastroenterologist when they recommend it. You'll take a PPI to reduce reflux and slow or rarely reverse Barrett's esophagus. They may also recommend aspirin because early evidence suggests it helps. Your GI doctor will see you often to look at your esophagus through a scope. They will remove tiny pieces of tissue called biopsies to see if Barrett's esophagus has changed to cancer. If they find high-grade Barrett's esophagus or cancer, scope-based treatments are available. The 3-step process of eating may help, especially if you have a stricture. Surgeons work with GI doctors to decide when to operate on Barrett's esophagus. If cancer develops, doctors remove the distal esophagus and pull the stomach upward into the chest—an esophagectomy and gastric pull through.

DIAGNOSIS: ESOPHAGEAL CANCER

Esophageal cancer is an abnormal growth of cells in the esophagus, causing food, pills, and liquid to get stuck during swallowing. These abnormal cells can invade lymph nodes. Advanced cancer travels through the bloodstream to other parts of the body—called metastases. Esophageal cancer is cancer. If you have esophageal cancer, you need a team to treat it. You need a gastroenterologist who probably found the tumor through a scope. You need a medical oncologist who is a cancer doctor. They treat cancer with medicines called chemotherapy and coordinate your cancer care among other doctors. You need a surgeon unless we discover incurable cancer. You need a radiation oncologist. They decide if you need radiation therapy to shrink the tumor before surgery. An ENT doctor may be part of your team. The surgeon you see may be a thoracic surgeon, a general surgeon, a cardiothoracic surgeon, or a surgical oncologist depending on the hospital. A radiologist is the physician who, through medical imaging, determines what stage the cancer is, usually with a PET-CT exam.

Cancer stage decides the treatment. Cancer stage describes what parts of the body are involved. Medical oncologists help you decide what treatment is best. Different cancer medications treat different cancer stages best, and the medical oncologist enables you to decide your best therapy. We treat esophageal cancer with cancer medications (aka, chemotherapy) and radiation therapy, typically at the same time. After chemotherapy and radiation therapy, they may do surgery.

During the operation, your surgeon removes the esophageal cancer and reconstructs your esophagus. They pull your stomach upward into your chest to connect with your remaining esophagus. That's most common. Sometimes, part of your colon takes the place of the esophagus. Your surgeon will guide you to your best option.

The 3-step approach to eating may be helpful before surgery, depending on how much the cancer blocks your esophagus. The 3-step approach may help after surgery.

We rarely use PPIs for esophageal cancer before surgery. After surgery, a PPI may help GERD.

Pro tip: If your medical oncologist can enroll you in a clinical trial, that's the best choice. Clinical trials compare the best treatment with a newer, potentially better, therapy. I tell family members to take part in clinical trials.

DIAGNOSIS: POST-RADIATION ESOPHAGITIS

Radiation destroys cancer cells in the esophagus. It also injures healthy parts of the esophagus, and doctors help with this injury. Post-radiation esophagitis is your normal esophagus reacting to radiation. If you have chest pain while eating or food gets stuck, talk to your radiation oncologist or medical oncologist. Treatments are available. Most patients treated for esophageal cancer go through a phase where they can't eat, or it's challenging.

If you can swallow food, the 3-step process may help.

Follow the advice of your radiation oncologist and medical oncologist and make sure they endorse this approach.

A PPI is not typically part of the therapy plan for post-radiation esophagitis. Surgery doesn't help esophagitis.

If radiation treatment succeeds, surgery may cure esophageal cancer and remove the inflamed esophagus at the same time.

POP QUIZ

Q. Which of the following is a precursor to esophageal cancer?

1. Gastroesophageal reflux disease (GERD).

2. Esophageal stricture.

3. Eosinophilic esophagitis.

4. Hiatal hernia.

5. Barrett's esophagus.

Answer: 5. Barrett's esophagus. Patients with Barrett's esophagus have a 0.1–0.5 percent chance per year their disease transforms to esophageal cancer. They MUST follow up with their doctor carefully.

TRANSFORMATION

There are many more diseases, syndromes, procedures, and surgeries I could cover. Chapter 12 explains the majority of problems of the average reader.

I did not discuss gastrostomy and jejunostomy tubes. If you need one, they are a blessing. My youngest daughter has had one since she was three months old. They allow patients to receive the nutrition they need to stay alive. I do hope, though, that this book empowers patients to collaborate more with their doctors and avoid these tubes if possible.

If you take nothing else from this final chapter, remember

Michelle's transformation. Michelle faced challenges in her life, like you. She struggled through emotional lows and celebrated highs. Esophagus attacks represent Michelle's latest struggle. Michelle's family supported her, and that helped her work through this problem. She stays on top of her disease. Michelle will succeed despite her esophagus challenge. You have inner strength like Michelle. Tap into it. You've worked to understand your esophagus problem. You will take care of it. You've come so far!

You must commit to examining your emotional basement or fear cave. Anger, frustration, uncertainty, isolation, pain, confusion, and denial are common roadblocks to progress. Know they sit in your path to healing. Face them. Sit with them. Journal. Talk with others. Meditate, reflect, and practice mindfulness training. Work through these emotions. As you do, they weaken their grasp on you. They stop running up the basement steps and crashing your party.

If you don't do the work and face these emotions, they wreak havoc in your life. Ask me how I know. I had emotional work to do after my four-month-old son, Ben, died. When Caroline was diagnosed with the same disease that killed Ben, feelings from my emotional basement kept popping up and causing problems.

Do the work. Or play emotional Whack-A-Mole in your mind and heart.

CONCLUSION

I've shared patient stories throughout this book to help you feel less alone and to give you role models for positive change. I celebrate each patient who achieves lifestyle changes to take care of their esophagus. Patients who treated their GERD, who see their doctors, who reschedule their meals. Patients who manage to lose weight or quit smoking. And of course, patients who find relief with the 3-step method for eating. I especially celebrate when patients succeeded by making enduring changes that forever improve their esophagus for the better. They'll never know it, but they could be saving themselves from a battle with an esophagus stricture or Barrett's esophagus.

You've come to the end of this book. You understand the esophagus. You know 99 percent of the time, your esophagus attack *isn't* from cancer. You know my three common-sense steps to eat with more confidence. Most patients figure this out after years or decades, but this book speeds up the learning curve. Esophagus attacks are a common problem, and in society, we talk little about it. Over-the-counter and prescription medicines help prevent this from worsening. With your doctor, you will fix this problem.

All this helps on your journey to eating more easily, more confidently, and with less anxiety.

Food getting stuck was a weakness for me. I was ashamed about it and didn't tell my wife for years. I worried about heart attacks and cancer. I faced this and learned about it. I transformed fear and weakness into a strength. Talking about my problem with patients with the same problem and sharing my common-sense solution inspired this book. I turned my pain, weakness, and shame into a book to help others.

You, too, can help others—promise three things. One, promise yourself to talk to your doctor if you haven't. Two, promise yourself to tell your loved ones and ask for their understanding. Three, chat with friends about this and support others who have this problem. Together we will remove the stigma people feel about esophagus attacks. Your pain and your experience will help someone else. My ten-year-old daughter read me a quote from Oprah Winfrey that nails this: "Turn your wounds into wisdom." Who knows, maybe "Esophagus-Friendly" will show up on restaurant menus like "Gluten-Free" or "Nut-Free?"

Please contact me if you have any comments, concerns, suggestions, or feedback. My email is douglakemd@gmail.com. I may not get back to you right away, and I cannot give medical advice over email, but I'd love to hear from you. Who knows, what works for you may help others. *Esophagus Attack!* second edition, may feature your ideas! Finally, share successes on social media. Use #EsophagusAttack, #Food-Stuck, #FoodIsFuel and #EatClean and draw others into the conversation. If you use Twitter, please include me (@ douglakemd).

Thank you for reading, and please be well!

NOTES

CHAPTER 2: MEDICAL SCHOOL FOR THE ESOPHAGUS: ANATOMY

The frequency of deglutition in man. Lear CS, Flanagan JB Jr, Moorres CF. Arch Oral Biol 1965; 10: 83-100.

Hiatal and Paraesophageal Hernias. Callaway JP, Vaezi MF. Clinical Gastroenterology and Hepatology Vol. 16, No. 6. P 810-813.

Palliative intubation of oesophagogastric neoplasms at fibreoptic endoscopy. Ogilvie AL, Dronfield MW, Ferguson R, Atkinson M. Gut. 1982; 23 (12): 1060–7.

Topography of normal and high-amplitude esophageal peristalsis. Clouse RE, Staiano A. Am J Physiol. 1993 Dec; 265 (6 Pt 1): G1098-1107.

CHAPTER 3: RESIDENCY FOR THE ESOPHAGUS: PRACTICAL APPLICATION

Esophageal Foreign Bodies and Obstruction in the Emergency Department Setting: An Evidence-Based Review. Long B, Koyfman A, Gottlieb M. J Emerg Med. 2019 May; 56 (5): 499-511.

The evolution of treatment and complications of esophageal food impaction. Schupack DA, Lenz CJ, Geno DM, et al. United European Gastroenterol J. 2019 05; 7 (4): 548-556.

Management of ingested foreign bodies and food impactions. ASGE Standards of Practice Committee, Ikenberry SO, Jue TL, Anderson MA, et al. Gastrointest Endosc. 2011 Jun; 73 (6): 1085-91.

CHAPTER 4: FELLOWSHIP FOR THE ESOPHAGUS: SPECIALIZATION

How I Approach Dysphagia. Kim JP, Kahrilas PJ. Curr Gastroenterol Rep. 2019 Aug 20; 21 (10): 49.

How to Approach a Patient with Eosinophilic Esophagitis. Hirano I. Gastroenterology. 2018 09; 155 (3): 601-606.

Limited value of alarm features in the diagnosis of upper gastrointestinal malignancy: systematic review and meta-analysis. Vakil N, Moayyedi P, Fennerty MB, Talley NJ. Gastroenterology. 2006 Aug; 131 (2): 390-401

"Use of a 13 mm barium tablet for analysis of potential esophageal stricture disease." Scott RL. (letter) AJR 2017; 208: [web] W196. Use of a 13 mm Barium Tablet for Analysis of Potential Esophageal Stricture Disease. Levine MS and Canon CL. American Journal of Roentgenology. 2017; 208: W197-W197.

CHAPTER 5: KNOW WHAT TO DO WHEN FOOD IS STUCK

Composition and Functions: A Comprehensive review. de Almeida PDV, Grégio AMT, Machado MÂN, et al. Saliva J Contemp Dent Pract 2008 March; (9) 3: 072-080.

Quantifying EGJ morphology and relaxation with high-resolution manometry: a study of seventy-five asymptomatic volunteers. Pandolfino JE, Ghosh SK, Zhang Q, et al. Am J Physiol Gastrointest Liver Physiol. 2006 May; 290 (5): G1033-40.

CHAPTER 7: EASY SOLIDS BEFORE DIFFICULT SOLIDS

The Art of Cookery in the Middle Ages (Studies in Anglo-Saxon History). Terence Scully. BOYE6; New edition, Sep 7, 1995.

Effect of aging on oral and swallowing function after meal consumption. Hiramatsu T, Kataoka H, Osaki M, Hagino H. Clin Interv Aging. 2015; 10: 229-35.

CHAPTER 9: LIFESTYLE CHANGES

Abdominal Compression by Waist Belt Aggravates Gastroesophageal Reflux, Primarily by Impairing Esophageal Clearance. Mitchell DR, Derakhshan MH, Wirz AA, et al. Gastroenterology. 2017 Jun; 152 (8): 1881-1888.

The adverse effect of chocolate on lower esophageal sphincter pressure. Wright LE, Castell DO. Am J Dig Dis. 1975; 20: 703-707.

Are Lifestyle Measures Effective in Patients with Gastroesophageal Reflux Disease? An Evidence-Based Approach. Kaltenbach T, Crockett S, Gerson LB. Arch Intern Med. 2006; 166: 965-971.

Association between coffee intake and GERD: A Meta-Analysis. Kim J, Oh SW, Myung SK, et al. Korean Meta-analysis (KORMA) Study Group. Dis Esophagus. 2014 May-Jun; 27 (4): 311-7.

Association between genetic variants and esophageal cancer
risk. Yue C, Li M, Da C, et al. Oncotarget. 2017 Jul 18; 8 (29):
47167-47174.

Interactions Between Genetic Variants and Environmental
Factors Affect Risk of Esophageal Adenocarcinoma and
Barrett's Esophagus. Dong J, Levine DM, Buas MF, et al. Clin
Gastroenterol Hepatol. 2018 Oct; 16 (10): 1598-1606.

Does physical activity protect against the development of
gastroesophageal reflux disease, Barrett's esophagus, and
esophageal adenocarcinoma? A review of the literature with a
meta-analysis. Lam S and Hart AR. Dis Esophagus. 2017 Nov
1; 30 (11): 1-10.

Early dinner reduces nocturnal gastric acidity. Duroux P,
Bauerfeind P, Emde C, et al. Gut. 1989 Aug; 30 (8): 1063-7.

The effect of chewing sugar-free gum on gastroesophageal reflux.
Moazzez R, Bartlett D, Anggiansah A. J Dent Res. 2005 Nov;
84 (11): 1062-5.

Effect of esomeprazole on nighttime heartburn and sleep
quality in patients with GERD: a randomized placebo-
controlled trial. Johnson DA, Orr WC, Crawley JA, et al. Am J
Gastroenterol 2005; 100: 1914 –1922.

Effect of high-fat, standard, and functional food meals on esophageal and gastric pH in patients with gastroesophageal reflux disease and healthy subjects. Fan WJ, Hou YT, Sun XH, et al. J Dig Dis. 2018 Nov; 19 (11): 664-673.

The effect of raw onions on acid reflux and reflux symptoms. Allen ML, Mellow MH, Robinson MG, Orr WC. Am J Gastroenterol. 1990 Apr; 85 (4): 377-80.

Effects of gastroesophageal reflux disease on sleep and outcomes. Mody R, Bolge SC, Kanna H, et al. Clin Gastroenterol Hepatol 2009; 7: 953–959.

Effects of Intermittent Fasting on Health, Aging and Disease NEJM 2019; 381: 2541-2551.

Effects of posture on gastroesophageal reflux. Stanciu C, Bennett JR. Digestion. 1977; 15: 104-109.

Epidemiology of gastroesophageal reflux disease: a general population-based study in Xi'an of Northwest China. Wang JH, Luo JY, Dong L, et a. World J Gastroenterol. 2004; 10: 1647-1651.

Food sensitivity in reflux esophagitis. Price SF, Smithson KW, Castell DO. Gastroenterology. 1978; 75: 240-243.

Gastroesophageal pressure gradients in gastroesophageal reflux disease: relations with hiatal hernia, body mass index, and esophageal acid exposure. de Vres DR, van Herwaarden MA, Smout AJ, et al. Am J Gastroenterol 2008; 103: 1349–1354.

Information on Genetic Variants Does Not Increase Identification of Individuals at Risk of Esophageal Adenocarcinoma Compared to Clinical Risk Factors. Kunzmann AT, Cañadas Garre M, Thrift AP, et al. Gastroenterology. 2019 Jan; 156 (1): 43-45.

Interactions Between Genetic Variants and Environmental Factors Affect Risk of Esophageal Adenocarcinoma and Barrett's Esophagus. Dong J, Levine DM, Buas MF, et al. Clin Gastroenterol Hepatol. 2018 Oct; 16 (10): 1598-1606.

Lack of effect of spearmint on lower oesophageal sphincter function and acid reflux in healthy volunteers. Bulat R, Fachnie U, Chaugan U, et al. Aliment Pharmacol Ther 1999; 13: 805-812.

Metabolic impacts of altering meal frequency and timing: Does when we eat matter? Hutchison AT, Heilbronn LK. Biochimie. 2016 May; 124: 187-197.

Mechanism of association between BMI and dysfunction of the gastroesophageal barrier in patients with normal endoscopy. Derakhshan MH, Robertson EV, Fletcher J, et al. Gut 2012; 61: 337–343.

Nocturnal reflux episodes following the administration of a standardized meal. Does timing matter? Piesman M, Hwang I, Maydonovitch C, Wong RK. Am J Gastroenterol. 2007 Oct; 102 (10): 2128-34.

Obesity: a challenge to esophagogastric junction integrity. Pandolfino JE, El-Serag HB, Zhang Q, et al. Gastroenterology 2006; 130: 639–649.

Obesity and estrogen as risk factors for gastroesophageal reflux symptoms. Nilsson M, Johnsen R, Ye W, et al. JAMA. 2003; 290: 66-72.

The pH of beverages in the United States. Reddy A, Norris DF, Momeni SS, et al. J Am Dent Assoc. 2016 Apr; 147 (4): 255-63.

Predictors of Heartburn During Sleep in a Large Prospective Cohort Study. Fass R, Quan SF, O'Connor GT, et al. CHEST 2005; 127: 1658–1666.

Relationship between body mass and gastroesophageal reflux symptoms: the Bristol Helicobacter Project. Murray L, Johnston B, Lane A, et al. Int J Epidemiol. 2003; 32: 645-650.

Relationship between sleep quality and pH monitoring findings in persons with gastroesophageal reflux disease. Dickman R, Green C, Fass SS, et al. J Clin Sleep Med 2007; 3: 505–513.

Relationship between upper gastrointestinal symptoms and lifestyle, psychosocial factors and comorbidity in the general population: results from the Domestic/International Gastroenterology Surveillance Study (DIGEST). Stanghellini V. Scand J Gastroenterol Suppl. 1999; 231: 29- 37.

Sleeping on a wedge diminishes exposure of the esophagus to refluxed acid. Hamilton JW, Boisen RJ, Yamamoto DT, et al. Dig Dis Sci. 1988; 33: 518-522.

Symptomatic gastroesophageal reflux: incidence and precipitating factors. Nebel OT, Fornes MF, Castell DO. Am J Dig Dis. 1976; 21: 953-956.

Symptoms of gastroesophageal reflux: prevalence, severity, duration and associated factors in a Spanish population. Diaz-Rubio M, Moreno Elola Olaso C, Rey E, et al. Aliment Pharmacol Ther. 2004; 19: 95-105.

Syndromic Surveillance for E-Cigarette, or Vaping, Product Use– Associated Lung Injury. Harnett KP, Kite-Powell A, Patel MT, et al. N Engl J Med 2020; 382: 766-772.

A systematic review of the definitions, prevalence, and response
to treatment of nocturnal gastroesophageal reflux disease.
Gerson LB, Fass R. Clin Gastroenterol Hepatol 2009; 7:
372–378.

Tobacco Smoking Cessation and Improved Gastroesophageal
Reflux: A Prospective Population-Based Cohort Study: The
HUNT Study. Ness-Jensen E, Lindam A, Lagergren J, et al.
Am J Gastroenterol 2014; 109: 171–177.

CHAPTER 10: MEDICATIONS

Comparison of the effects of immediate-release omeprazole
oral suspension, delayed-release lansoprazole capsules and
delayed-release esomeprazole capsules on nocturnal gastric
acidity after bedtime dosing in patients with night-time
GERD symptoms. Katz PO, Koch FK, Ballard ED, et al.
Aliment Pharmacol There 2007; 25: 197-205.

Gastroesophageal reflux disease during pregnancy. Katz PO,
Castell DO. Gastroenterol Clin 1998; 27: 153-167.

On-demand therapy for gastroesophageal reflux disease. Metz
DC, Inadomi JM, Howden CW, et al. Am J Gastroenterol
2007; 102: 642-653.

Overprescribing PPIs: Time for a hospital antacid policy on
Clostridium difficile. Thachil J. BMJ 2008; 336: 109.

Proton pump inhibitor use and the risk for community-acquired pneumonia. Sarkar M, Hennessy S, Yang YX. Ann Intern Med 2008; 149: 391-398.

Ranitidine versus cimetidine in the healing of erosive esophagitis. McCarty-Dawson D, Sue So, Morrill B, et al. Clin There 1996; 18: 1150-1160.

Role of gastric acid suppression in the treatment of gastroesophageal reflux disease. Bell MJV, Hunt RH. Gut 1992; 33: 118-124.

Step-down management of gastroesophageal reflux disease. Inadomi JM, Jamal R, Murata GH, et al. Gastroenterology 2001; 121: 1095-1100.

Use of proton pump inhibitors and the risk of community-acquired pneumonia: A population-based case control study. Ulmez SE, Holm, A, Frederiksen H, et al. Arch Intern Med 2007; 102: 2047-2056.

Use of proton pump inhibitors and risk of osteoporosis-related fractures. Targownik LE, Lix LM, Merge CJ. CMAJ 2008; 179: 319-326.

CHAPTER 12: DIAGNOSES ASSOCIATED WITH ESOPHAGUS ATTACKS

Approaches and Challenges to Management of Pediatric and
Adult Patients with Eosinophilic Esophagitis. Hirano I,
Furuta GT. Gastroenterology. 2020 Mar; 158 (4): 840-851.

Association of Acute Gastroesophageal Reflux Disease with
Esophageal Histologic Changes. Dunbar KB, Agoston AT,
Odze, RD, et al. JAMA 2016; 315 (19): 2104-2112.

Controversies in the management of caustic ingestion injury: an
evidence-based review. Bird JH, Kumar S, Paul C, Ramsden
JD. Clin Otolaryngol. 2017 Jun; 42 (3): 701-708.

Endoscopic incisional therapy for benign esophageal strictures:
Technique and results. Samanta J, Dhaka. N, Sinha SK,
Kochhar R. World J Gastrointest Endosc. 2015 Dec 25; 7 (19):
1318-26.

Efficacy of a 4-Food Elimination Diet for Children with
Eosinophilic Esophagitis. Kagalwalla AF, Wechsler JB,
Amsden K, et al. Clinical Gastroenterology and Hepatology
2017; 15: 1698-1707.

Epidemiology and Natural History of Eosinophilic Esophagitis.
Dellon ES, Hirano I. Gastroenterology. 2018 01; 154 (2): 319-332.
e3.

Four-food group elimination diet for adult eosinophilic
esophagitis: A prospective multicenter study. Molina-Infante J,
Arias A, Barrio J, et al. American Academy of Allergy, Asthma,
& Immunology 2014; 134: 1093-1099.

How to Approach a Patient with Eosinophilic Esophagitis.
Hirano I. Gastroenterology. 2018 09; 155 (3): 601-606.

A New Paradigm for GERD Pathogenesis. Not Acid Injury,
but cytokine-mediated inflammation driven by HIF-2a: a
potential role for targeting HIF-2a to prevent and treat reflux
esophagitis. Souza RF, Bayeh L, Spechler SJ, et al. Current
Opinion in Pharmacology 2017; 37: 93-99.

Plastic and biodegradable stents for complex and refractory
benign esophageal strictures. Ham YH, Kim GH. Clin Endosc.
2014 Jul; 47 (4): 295-300.

The refractory and the recurrent esophageal stricture: a
definition. Kochman ML, McClave SA, Boyce HW.
Gastrointest Endosc. 2005; 62D3]: 474–5.

Refractory esophageal strictures: what to do when dilation
fails. van Boeckel PG, Siersema PD. Curr Treat Options
Gastroenterol. 2015 Mar; 13 (1): 47-58.

The Relationship Between Hiatal Hernia and Cricopharyngeus
Muscle Dysfunction. Nativ-Zeltzer N, Rameau A, Kuhn MA,
et al. Dysphagia. 2019 Jun; 34 (3): 391-396.

Rule of three for esophageal dilation: like the tortoise versus
the rabbit, low and slow is our friend and our patients' win.
Richter, JE. Gastrointest Endosc. 2017 Feb; 85 (2): 338-339.

Will a Proton Pump Inhibitor and an Aspirin Keep the Doctor
Away for Patients with Barrett's Esophagus? Fitzgerald RC,
Corley DA. Gastroenterology. 2019 Apr; 156 (5): 1228-1231.

ACKNOWLEDGMENTS

Thank you to my amazing wife, Maleia. You're shuttling in and out of Boston Children's with Caroline. I'm shuttling Grace and Charlotte to and from Boston every chance we had. Our lives were a cacophony, and I proposed writing a book? Three years later, I finished a ten-chapter dumpster-fire rough draft. I proposed rewriting it and your answer? More support. Thank you for loving me and supporting me through this and so much more.

A very special thank you to the world's best eleven-year-old editor and cover illustrator, Grace Lake! When you said, "Daddy, the medical stuff isn't that great, but your stories kept me reading," it forever changed my approach to the book. Thank you, G.

Love-A-Lot Charlotte! You snapped pictures of me in different ties and shirts for the author portrait. You helped me pick out the best shirt and tie. This book wouldn't be here without your constant love and support. You are our middle daughter. You're the rock of our family. I love and appreciate you.

Caroline Bear-O-Line, this book wouldn't be here without you. Our journey with you to Boston inspired this book. I'd been in hospitals since middle school. I'd seen patients struggle. I never felt it in my heart as I did with Ben and, later, you. When we arrived to the BCH cardiac ICU and Dr. Kheir and fellows, residents, nurses, technologists and countless others helped you, something new lit inside me. When Dr. Baird opened up your heart and fixed it, something in my heart got fixed. I found inspiration to help others that sprang from me and wouldn't stop. Some call it a quantum change. Thank you to you and to sweet Ben.

Thank you, Mom and Dad, for your unending support, love and wisdom. You shaped, motivated, and supported me. From "Doug Days" as a child to multiple graduations, a wedding, and four births, you've been there. I know you're both proud. I love you.

My extended family, thank you. Both the Lake and Rome families have lifted us up with prayer and support for years. You've helped us in so many ways that led to this book emerging. Trips to Boston, prayer teams, unexpected trips to Ames, lifting us. Your love means so much to us. Thank you!

A shout-out to Our Caring Bridge family, Fr. Jim Secora, and the St. Cecilia community in Ames. You've read our blog posts, lifted us in prayer, and supported our family in so many ways. You raised an amazing amount of money when Caroline first got sick. Your love, from Ames and around our world, helped so much.

The Medical University of South Carolina radiology residency took a chance on a guy from Kansas. Thank you for investing thousands of hours in my education, leadership, and development. I cannot name the hundreds of smiling faces from the Lowcountry who help make Charleston "The Friendliest City." Your spirit of giving inspired this book.

Thank you, Dr. Schabel. You give more than any mentor I've ever had. I ask for a blurb and you return a two-page edit and write a book foreword! Your love for your resident and student family is obvious. Thank you.

Stanford Radiology took an even bigger chance on me as their clinical MRI fellow for a year. My head learned so much at Stanford, but my heart learned more. After all, it is Leland Stanford Junior University. Stanford Radiology demonstrates grace weathering the loss of so many fantastic colleagues. Many helped me over the years. Like MUSC, I cannot begin to name names. Thank you.

Thank you Boston Children's Hospital, the cardiology division, and especially the pulmonary vein stenosis team. You saved Caroline's life. Literally. Time and again. You also saved our family. I can't imagine if we had returned from Boston without Caroline. You push back against a lethal disease and dedicate your lives to the fight. You inspired me to share my story with patients and inspired this book. Kathy Jenkins, Ryan Callahan, Christina Ireland, Jim Lock, John Kheir, Chris Baird, Jessica Rosenhaus Traniello and so many others—thank you.

Thank you, Andrew Perry and Brian Dieter. Your guidance and leadership helped me develop as a medical leader. I appreciate your support for me and my family.

Thank you, McFarland Clinic Radiology extended family. You supported my family when we left for a month with Caroline when she was sick. Your grace amid challenges like the June 2016 car accident with Deb Thompson and Dr. Skinner was amazing.

Huge thank you to Dr. Bryan Graveline. Looking back, I can't believe I asked you to wade through my dumpster fire rough draft. You're a great colleague and our patients are so lucky to have you at McFarland Clinic.

I have so much appreciation for my McFarland physician team, especially our GI docs, ENTs, general surgeons, and medical oncologists. There are too many of you to name, but you've taught me so much about your areas of expertise. I'm blessed to work on an exceptional team.

To Shelley Goecke, for advising me early in the project, supporting the project along the way, and fielding my random marketing and strategy questions.

Hal Clifford and Emily Gindlesparger, you locked in my outline. Your one-two punch on the weekly Scribe support calls is exceptional. Scribe struck gold on you! Your support for authors is unmatched and your emotional intelligence is off the charts.

Thank you, Tucker Max. The man I met in Austin has little in common with the storyteller from IHTSBIH. Your wisdom about writing, publishing, marketing, and emotional intelligence is phenomenal. Under your leadership, Scribe Media pioneered a third pathway to publishing a book. You married self-publishing with decades of traditional publishing experience and knowledge. You're helping average people like me write books to help the world. Fantastic!

Special thanks to Ellie Cole, my publishing manager, for always having something upbeat no matter the scenario. You kept this train on the tracks and on time. A month of manuscript edits gone? Nothing but calm suggestions. Derecho inland hurricane knocks out my internet for two weeks during editing? How can Scribe help, Doug? Phenomenal.

Colleen Kapklein, I don't know how you're both an editor and a neurosurgeon, but you opened my head, figured out what I meant to write, and wrote it better. The reader benefits from your years of expertise. Wow and thank you!

Please judge "Esophagus Attack!" by its cover! Thank you, Rachael Brandenburg, for wading through my verbal and written descriptions of my ideal book cover. Then, you executed it at a high level and kept us from gutter ideas that wouldn't work. Outstanding work!

If the title caused you to take a second look at the book, Chas Hoppe is the reason. Thank you Chas for helping me come up with the perfect title!

Dan McClanahan, wow! Thank you for wading through my long e-mails and crafting a stunning author portrait. Your work blesses Ames and Central Iowa.

Thank you to Jill Paulus and Max Oxygen Crossfit family for their unending support of my family. You've helped in obvious and less obvious ways along my author journey. I'm so blessed to be part of a fantastic Crossfit family. Thank you!

Jeanne, Rod, Teri, Mark, Jim, Mary, Alice, Amanda, Susan, Shanea, Paige, Morgan, Allie, Audrey, Lexie, Becca and many others, thank you. You came into our home and treated my girls like your own. My girls blossomed under your care and attention. You helped me work through this project to help others. Thank you!

"Jesus heard them and answered, 'Healthy people don't need a doctor, but sick people do.' Go and learn what the Scriptures mean when they say, 'Instead of offering sacrifices to me, I want you to be merciful to others.' I didn't come to invite good people to be my followers. I came to invite sinners." Matthew 9: 12-13. We may call our Higher Power by different names around our world, but thank you God and Jesus for helping me be a better physician. Fr. Richard Rohr, thank you for casting light among shadows and helping me more than you'll ever know.

ABOUT THE AUTHOR

DR. DOUG LAKE practices radiology at the McFarland Clinic PC in Ames, Iowa, and maintains a part-time Adjunct Clinical Assistant Professor position in Radiology at Stanford.

He holds degrees from Loyola University Chicago and the University of Kansas, and he was a Chief Radiology Resident at the Medical University of South Carolina and a clinical MRI fellow at Stanford.

Dr. Lake is passionate about public health, and he has spoken at the White House as an advocate for better insurance options. Dr. Lake and his wife, Maleia, also founded the Home for Hope, a housing choice for families with children with pulmonary vein stenosis.

CPSIA information can be obtained
at www.ICGtesting.com
Printed in the USA
LVHW031926030221
678261LV00026B/332

9 781544 516974